Innate Immunity - New Perspectives and Therapeutic Opportunities

Edited by Ahmed Lasfar

Published in London, United Kingdom

Innate Immunity - New Perspectives and Therapeutic Opportunities
http://dx.doi.org/10.5772/intechopen.111143
Edited by Ahmed Lasfar

Contributors
Ali A. Alyahawi, Ali Haider Mohammed, Atteaya Zaman, B. Pushpa, Bassam Abdul Rasool Hassan, Boyuan Shen, Hajra Fayyaz, Imran Ullah, J. Saminathan, Mohammed AW. Almorish, Muhammad Hasnain Murtaza, R.A. Shanmugha Priya, Saeid Besharati, Ushus S. Kumar, Waheed Rafiq, Xiang Zhou, Yinghong He, Zonghai Chen

First published in London, United Kingdom, 2025 by IntechOpen
IntechOpen is the global imprint of INTECHOPEN LIMITED, registered in England and Wales, registration number: 11086078, 167-169 Great Portland Street, London, W1W 5PF, United Kingdom

For EU product safety concerns: IN TECH d.o.o., Prolaz Marije Krucifikse Kozulić 3, 51000 Rijeka, Croatia, info@intechopen.com or visit our website at intechopen.com.

British Library Cataloguing-in-Publication Data
A catalogue record for this book is available from the British Library

Innate Immunity - New Perspectives and Therapeutic Opportunities
Edited by Ahmed Lasfar
p. cm.
Print ISBN 978-1-83634-128-4
Online ISBN 978-1-83634-127-7
eBook (PDF) ISBN 978-1-83634-129-1

Meet the editor

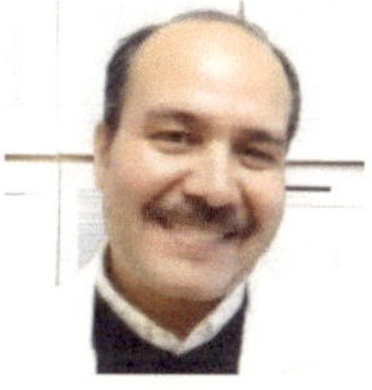

Dr. Lasfar is a full member of the Rutgers-Cancer Institute of New Jersey and a faculty member of Rutgers University. He's a leading cancer immunologist, a principal investigator, a consultant on drugs and an editor of several books and journals. His research is focused on breast cancer, liver cancer and melanoma. His laboratory is funded by the National Institute of Health and other sources. Dr. Lasfar graduated in Medical and Applied Science from Paris Rene Descartes University in France. He completed his doctoral specialty in Immunology at Paris Diderot University and his postdoctoral training in Cancer Immunology at Robert Wood Johnson Medical School, New Jersey.

Contents

Preface

Innate immunity is the first line of defense against harmful pathogens and the emergence of tumor cells in the body. Innate immunity functions through its anatomical and cellular components, particularly involving various factors and cytokines crucial to inflammatory processes.

In contrast to adaptive immunity, innate immunity is inherited and acts quickly to evade pathogens and cancer cells. Innate immunity can recognize and eliminate any dangers or, in many situations, unclench the adaptive immunity, which consists of more specific and robust immunity.

Innate immunity is promoted by activating various immune cells, such as basophils, neutrophils and natural killer cells. Although the mechanisms of immune cell activation are distinct, specific cytokines are released and lead to inflammation. TNF, IL-1 and type I with type III interferons orchestrate the inflammatory process to eliminate foreign substances. However, in some patients, the inflammation exacerbates autoimmune diseases.

Dysfunctions in innate immunity lead not only to frequent infectious diseases but also to the promotion of cancer and inflammation. Our current understanding at the molecular levels of many facets of innate immunity has contributed to the elaboration of critical therapeutic strategies that are crucial in alleviating and saving many patients' lives. Those points are addressed in this book.

Significant efforts and collaborations with leading experts in this field contributed to achieving this high-quality book with rich and authentic information. We thank all the contributors for sharing their expertise, expressing their specific visions, and bringing new hopes to patients suffering from immune dysfunctions and inflammatory diseases. Readers will appreciate the novelty and reliability of the information this book delivers.

Ahmed Lasfar
Full Member at Rutgers-New Jersey Cancer Institute,
Faculty Member of Ernest Mario School of Pharmacy,
Department of Pharmacology and Toxicology,
Rutgers University,
Piscataway, New Jersey, USA

Section 1

Role of Innate Immunity in Infection Diseases

Chapter 1

Immunosuppression in Infectious Diseases: Causes and Effects

Hajra Fayyaz, Atteaya Zaman, Waheed Rafiq, Muhammad Hasnain Murtaza and Imran Ullah

Abstract

Immunosuppression is the reduction in the normal immune system. This suppression weakens the activation and functioning of the immune system, making individuals more susceptible to infections. By understanding immunosuppression, the recognition, management, and treatment of infectious diseases can be achieved. Generally, immunosuppression is associated with the outcome of a disease (primary or secondary immunodeficiencies). Currently, a large population is facing immunosuppression due to the exposure of therapeutic drugs. These medications modulate the immune system and effectively manage immune-related diseases, but they also increase the chance of infections. The clinical picture of infectious diseases in immune-suppressed individuals differs from the immune-competent, making the diagnosis challenging. Therefore, recognition and management of immunosuppression are necessary for preventing and curing the affected population. Herein, we will discuss an overview of immunosuppression and its role in infectious diseases, how immune cells and molecules work together to combat pathogens, the causes of immunosuppression (particularly primary immunodeficiency), and its clinical, diagnostic, and effects on human health.

Keywords: primary immunodeficiency, secondary immunodeficiency, immunosuppression, tolerance, autoimmunity

1. Introduction

Human defense from infection relies on a complex integrated system consisting of physical barriers, chemical barriers, and an immune system. The immune system comprises two compartments, innate and adaptive immunity, which have different modes of action [1]. Innate immunity is the first line of defense for fighting against pathogens. This immune response is rapid (minutes or hours); however, the response is not improved on repeated exposure, showing no immunologic memory. On the other hand, adaptative/acquired immunity is antigen-dependent and antigen-specific, associated with a delay in antigen exposure, and shows a maximum response. An important feature of immunity is memory, which allows the host to mount a faster and more effective immune response after exposure to an antigen. Innate immunity and adaptative immunity are not a combination of the host's defenses, they are complete and defects in any of the systems can lead to inappropriate responses [1, 2].

The innate immune system's constituents (macrophages, natural killers, neutrophils, and complement systems) identify foreign antigens by their respective receptors encoded by germline genes. These receptors bind with pathogen-associated molecular patterns (PAMPs), features shared by a variety of pathogens, and initiate a signaling cascade by activating the transcription factors involved in the expression of pro-inflammatory genes [3]. The adaptive immune system consists of B and T lymphocytes that identify the antigen by receptors made from the rearrangement of gene segments, and each lymphocyte has a specific and unique antigen-binding receptor. The B-cells have antigen-specific immunoglobulin receptors on their cell membrane. The binding of antigen with immunoglobulin results in the clone of progeny B-cells with identical specificity. These clone cells differentiate into plasma cells and secrete different immunoglobulins (IgG, IgM, IgA, IgD, or IgE). T-cells are important regulators of cell-mediated immunity. Like B-cells, T-cells also have specific antigenic binding sites, and the various regulatory functions of T-cells are achieved by lymphocyte subpopulations [3]. The continuous advancement in the current understanding of the immune system and how it regulates and functions to protect the human body from any infection requires an in-depth review.

2. Immune-mediated disorders

Immune-mediated disorders include a wide variety of illnesses characterized by dysfunction in the normal immune response. Most of these diseases are complex and are believed to occur due to genetic (primary) and environmental/medication factors (secondary) causing immunosuppression [4].

2.1 Infectious diseases

An important function of the immune system is to control the infection caused by pathogens (non-self) while maintaining immune tolerance to self-antigens. Infectious diseases are caused by different pathogens (bacteria, viruses, and fungi that infect the host body), and are increasing mortality worldwide [2]. For several years, many people considered Koch's postulates, which implied that virulence traits are specifically determined by the type of pathogen. However, current advancements in molecular biology reveal that host (human) genes play a main role in infection, collectively with environmental variables [5, 6]. Several genes are involved in the infection mechanism, and one of the genes that is associated with infectious disease and the immune system is the natural-resistance-associated macrophage protein (NRAMP1) which encodes an integral protein expressed in macrophages and monocytes. The region is considered a susceptibility locus for increasing the infection when infected by certain strains of Salmonella spp., Mycobacterium tuberculosis, and Mycobacterium bovis [7]. Moreover, it has also been proposed that functional variants of cluster of differentiation (CD32) are linked with the development of invasive encapsulated bacterial infections. Conclusively, one of the causes of immunosuppression is infectious disease (specifically viral disease), which impairs the development of lymphoid organs or dysregulates the function of lymphocytes [8].

2.2 Immunodeficiencies

Deficiency of lymphocytes (B- and T-cells) or immunoglobulin due to genetic abnormalities, disease, surgical events, or other reasons can reduce the host immunity, leading to immunosuppression. Collectively, any dysfunction in any of the components of the immune system results in immunodeficiency [9]. These can be genetic or intrinsic causes, such as defects in the elements of lymphoid cells, abnormal cellular differentiation, or acquired causes (viral infection) [10]. In clinical prospect, the immunity deficiency is explained as a pronounced susceptibility to pathogenic and opportunistic organisms that are hard to treat, and with the increase in infection there would be an increase in the risk of cancer, autoimmune disorders, and allergy [11]. These defects are represented as primary immunodeficiency diseases (PIDD) and secondary immunodeficiency diseases (SIDD). PIDD are inborn errors with a wide range of clinical presentations, notably recurrent and frequently life-threatening infections. The errors manifest early in life, ranging from microbial susceptibility to allergy, autoimmune disease, and lymphoproliferation. SIDD is defined as a disease affecting the immune system of the host by a stimulator that arises outside of the immune system and is often not restricted to immune elements [10, 11]. Even though more than 400 genes are defined as causing PIDDs, approximately 50–60% of the underlying genes are still unknown, and for this, next-generation sequencing (NGS) studies are largely contributing to identifying these unknown genes causing PIDDs [12]. An updated list of PIDD-causing genes and diseases is available on the webpage of the European Society for Immunodeficiencies (ESID) [13]. Herein, we have specifically discussed the observed immunological consequences and immunosuppression caused by PIDD.

2.2.1 Genetic defect in lymphoid cells

The most profound form of immunodeficiency is a group of heterogeneous disorders named severe combined immunodeficiency (SCID) that is characterized by abnormalities in both the T-cell and B-cell [14]. The defect occurs at the level of hematopoietic stem cells and leads to the virtual absence of T-cells, B-cells, and neutrophils. In the case of SCID, all components of the innate immune system are intact, even though severe combined immunodeficiency causes an absence or reduction of humoral and cell-mediated adaptive immunity. This group of disorders is almost always caused by defects in the T lymphocyte and affects both cellular and humoral immunity because of the essential role of CD4 T-cells. The growth and differentiation of B lymphocytes, as well as the growth and differentiation of T-cells, can be affected by the absence of CD4 T-cells [14, 15]. Affected children have severe deficiencies in all T lymphocyte subsets. The peripheral blood may or may not have normal numbers of B-cells. The affected children are unable to make antibody responses to vaccines or infections because of a lack of differentiation into plasma cells. Within the first few months of life, infants with SCID often become sick. Due to the immunosuppression caused by the deficiency of lymphocytes, the patients are frequently susceptible to microbial pathogens, including infections caused by enteroviruses and encapsulated bacteria. Additionally, they are at risk of a greater variety of viruses. Adenovirus, rotavirus, varicella-zoster virus (VZV), cytomegalovirus (CMV), respiratory syncytial virus (RSV), and other varied pathogens result in chronic infections. Fungal infections (aspergillosis and candidiasis) are challenging in SCID patients because the lack of CD4 T-lymphocytes results in no production of interferons necessary for the death of phagocytic cells. Opportunistic infections like Mycobacterium avium intracellulare, Pneumocystis jirovecii, and Mycobacterium bovis Bacille Calmette-Guerin (BCG) from vaccination can also infect SCID patients [16]. Currently, most of these infections can be cured while the underlying immunodeficiency is completely treated with a bone marrow transplant [17].

Several genetic defects have been identified in SCID patients with variable clinical manifestations. It is observed that the SCID patients either have pathogenic variants in the SCID-associated gene or a reduction in the proliferation of T-cells is detected in the presence of certain mitogens [18]. The genetic diagnosis of SCID is necessary for confirmation of clinical diagnosis and molecular pathways, which ultimately will be helpful in genetic counseling, and treatment. A summary of the genetic defects causing SCID is given in **Table 1**.

2.2.2 Genetic defects involve impaired differentiation of lymphoid cells

Common variable immunodeficiency (CVID) comprises a group of heterogeneous disorders that are characterized by impaired antibody responses and hypogammaglobulinemia. Furthermore, some immunologic abnormalities are variably expressed in patients such as T-cell dysregulation and autoimmune diseases [19]. Most patients manifest symptoms after the first decade of their lives, while some are present in their early childhood. CVID is linked with a high incidence of infections caused by encapsulated organisms and reduced secretion of immunoglobulins. In most patients, recurrent pneumonia, sinusitis, and/or bronchitis are predominant, and these

Type of SCID	**Involved gene/s**
Artemis SCID	*DCLRE1C*
X-linked SCID	*IL2R gamma*
Adenosine deaminase deficiency SCID	*ADA*
Cernunnos-XLF deficiency SCID	*NHEJ1*
CD3 complex component deficiency SCID	*CD3D, CD3E, CD247*
IL7R deficiency SCID	*IL7R alpha*
DNA ligase 4 deficiency SCID	*LIG4*
Coronin-1A deficiency SCID	*CORO1A*
JAK3 deficiency SCID	*JAK3*
Reticular dysgenesis SCID	*AK2*
LAT deficiency SCID	*LAT*
DNA-PKCS deficiency SCID	*PRKDC*
CD45 deficiency SCID	*PTPRC*
RAG1 and RAG2 deficiency SCID	*RAG1, RAG2*
Leaky SCID	*RAG1, RAG2* and some other genes
Omenn syndrome	*RAG1, RAG2*

Table 1.
Types of severe combined immunodeficiency and involved genes.

conditions ultimately develop chronic pulmonary dysfunction. Most of the detected pathogens causing respiratory tract infections are encapsulated bacteria, and about 60% of CVID patients have chronic diarrhea [20]. Literature shows that a broad range of immunologic abnormalities can give rise to different clinical presentations of CVID. The genetic mutation causing CVID impairs the functionality of the lymphocytes and leads to immunosuppression, as summarized in **Table 2**. For instance, genetic investigations have shown mutations in the different genes causing different subtypes of CVID, such as X-linked agammaglobulinemia (XLA) (defect in the Btk gene) [21], X-linked lymphoproliferative disease (SH2D1A defect) [22], and in some individuals, defects in activated T-cell stimulator (ICOS) have been previously identified. Such analyses are anticipated to aid in the definition of subgroups of CVID patients with varying presentations and prognostic factors and might result in new therapeutic approaches.

X-linked agammaglobulinemia (XLA) is a disorder of humoral immunity that is manifested by the early onset of recurrent infections. *S. aureus*, *S. pneumoniae*, and *H. influenzae* are very frequently bacterial pathogens, and groups of viruses (polioviruses, enteric cytopathogenic human orphan [ECHO], and coxsackie) are likely to cause meningoencephalitis, chronic diarrhea, pneumonitis, sinusitis, otitis media, and hepatitis in XLA patients [21]. Shreds of evidence showed that the defect occurs at the transition level from pre-B-cell to mature B-cell. Therefore, the patients with this disorder have low concentrations of immunoglobulin (panhypogammaglobulinemia) except IgE. The individuals also lack circulating B-lymphocytes and plasma cells. However, other components of the immune system and the thymus are normal.

Phenotype	Genetic defect
NF-κB1 deficiency	*NFKB1*
NF-κB2 deficiency	*NFKB2*
IKAROS deficiency	*IKAROS*
CD21 deficiency	*CD21*
STAT3 hyperactivity	*STAT3*
APDS 1 and APDS 2	*PIK3CD* *PIK3R1*
IRF2BP2 deficiency	*IRF2BP2*
CTLA-4 deficiency	*CTLA4*
LRBA deficiency	*LRBA*
ICOS deficiency	*ICOS*
TACI defect BAFF-R defect	*TNFRSF13B*
CD81 deficiency	*CD81*
X-linked agammaglobulinemia	Btk
Ataxia-telangiectasia.	ATM
Selective IgA deficiency	Genetic defect not well-defined
DiGeorge syndrome	Deletion of 22q11. 2

Table 2.
Genetic defects associated with the CVID-phenotype.

Initially, patients with XLA are protected by the presence of maternal IgG for the first few months of life. Subsequently, recurrent and chronic infections are the major clinical phenotypes of XLA [23].

Thymic hypoplasia (DiGeorge syndrome) is a condition with dysregulation in the development of T-cells. Patients have increased susceptibility to diarrhea, recurrent pneumonia, and sinusitis, and the frequent infections are mostly caused by protozoa and *Candida albicans*. The immunological profile showed a normal count of absolute lymphocyte count, but with a decreased percentage of T-lymphocytes and an increased percentage of B-lymphocytes with normal B-cell function. A decreased count of T-cells leads to a markable decrease in T-cell-mediated functions and collectively leads to immunodeficiency, as T-cells are important for activating the immune responses in cases of the most antigens. This deficiency suppresses the host immune system, and the patient suffers from recurrent infections [24]. Currently, fetal thymus transplantation results in the regaining of T-cell function, hence also suggesting that deficiency in thymic hormones might be a reason for this disease [25].

Another condition caused by the impaired function of both B and T lymphocytes is ataxia-telangiectasia. It is associated with repeated sinopulmonary infections and an increased occurrence of malignancies such as lymphoreticular tumors. The noticeable abnormality in the B-cell is the deficiency of IgA or/and IgE. The B lymphocytes express IgA on their surface, indicating that the defect would be at the level of differentiation rather than synthesis [26].

Another immunodeficiency caused by the defect in humoral immunity is selective IgA deficiency. The disease is manifested by the patient having a serum IgA level of less than 7 mg/dL, along with normal levels of other immunoglobulin, and a normal cell-mediated immune response. Since IgA is the primary secretory immunoglobulin, most infections in affected individuals develop on mucosal surfaces. Meningitis and bacterial sepsis are uncommon, while otitis media, pneumonia, sinusitis, bronchitis, and diarrhea are the most frequent phenotypes. Furthermore, IgA deficiency is linked with an enhanced risk of carcinoma, allergies, and autoimmune disorders. In most patients, a defect in the B-lymphocyte results in impairment of the transition of IgA-expressing B-cells into plasma cells that synthesize and secrete functional IgA [27].

2.2.3 Defect-causing neutrophilic phagocyte disorders

Neutrophils are short-lived cells that are involved in the elimination of different types of microorganisms. Dysfunction in the chemotaxis and phagocytosis increase susceptibility to opportunistic infections caused by bacteria, while patients do not experience infections caused by protozoa or viruses. Dysfunction in neutrophils is divided into two defects, intrinsic and extrinsic [28].

2.2.3.1 Intrinsic defects

In chronic granulomatous disease (CGD), the NADPH oxidase-dependent respiratory burst system of phagocytic cells is defective, resulting in intracellular killing. In CGD, the organisms causing infection are almost all catalase producers (Serratia marscens, *Staphylococcus aureus*, and Aspergillus). The frequent sites of infection in CGD patients are the skin, lymph nodes, lungs, perianal area, and gingivae. The phagocytic cell, which has live intracellular organisms, moves to reticuloendothelial tissues, that is, the spleen and liver, which results in sometimes large abscesses [29].

Chediak-Higashi syndrome (CHS) is a multisystem disorder due to a defect in the function of the neutrophilic microtubule. Primarily, this dysregulation is because of the inability of phagosomes and lysosomes to fuse after the ingestion of microorganisms. The dysfunction of the lysosomal trafficking regulator gene (LYST) affects the lysosomal trafficking function, hence increasing the incidence of pyogenic infections [30]. CHS is characterized by profound immunodeficiency with severe neutropenia, anemia, thrombocytopenia, progressive neuropathy, and recurrent skin and respiratory tract infections.

Currently, about 15 genes are reported and are known to be contributing to congenital neutropenia (**Table 3**).

2.2.3.2 Extrinsic defects

There are several extrinsic defects causing dysfunction in neutrophils and are related to decreased opsonization or leucopenia, abnormal chemotaxis, or the administration of drugs. Generally, when the neutrophilic count reduces to a critical level of ~1000/μl, the host system is likely to be infected by infection. Leukopenia is commonly induced by drugs. Anti-inflammatory drugs, that is, corticosteroids, induce dysregulation in neutrophil adherence and migration, leading to a deficiency in neutrophils functionality. Another mechanism is autoimmune neutropenia, which results in the deletion of neutrophils through the antibody-dependent lymphocyte-mediated cytotoxicity (ADCC) pathway. In drug-induced immune neutrophenia, the cells may absorb drug-antibody immune complexes, which may result in neutrophil destruction via an innocent bystander mechanism [28].

2.2.4 Disorders of the complement system

Distribution in the activation of C3 by the classical pathway cause the deficiency/dysregulation of C1q, C1r, C1s, C2, C3, or C4 proteins due to abnormalities in their respective genes. These disorders are associated with sepsis and other vascular

Phenotype	**Genetic defect**
Cyclic neutropenia	*ELANE*
Severe congenital neutropenia	*GFI1, WAS*
Wart hypogammaglobulinemia immunodeficiency myelokathexis (WHIM) syndrome	*CXCR4*
Kostmann' disease	*HAX1*
CSF3R deficiency	*CSF3R*
IRAK 4 deficiency	*IRAK 4*
Chediak-Higashi syndrome	*LYST*
Chronic granulomatous disease	*CYBA, CYBB, NCF1, NCF2, NCF4*
G6PC3 deficiency	*G6PC3*
VPS45 deficiency	*VPS45*

Table 3.
Genetic defects causing congenital neutrophilic phagocyte disorders.

diseases and bloodstream infections. The most frequent pathogens during these disorders are *Streptococcus pneumoniae, Haemophilus influenzae*, Enterobacteriaceae, Neisseria meningitidis, and staphylococci. Patients with deficiencies in the complement system are more susceptible to systemic lupus erythematosus (SLP), allergy, and autoallergic disease and even have an increased risk of malignancy. Recurrent infections caused by the same pathogen or with organisms having low pathogenicity and showing an incomplete response to suitable antibiotics are indicative of impaired immunity [31].

2.3 Autoimmune disorders

During the development of B- and T-cells, self-reactive B- and T-cells are removed via apoptosis, however, few reactive cells escape into the periphery. The human immune system modulates several mechanisms to ensure that these self-reactive cells remain unresponsive toward self-antigens. One of the tolerance mechanisms is central tolerance, in which active T-cells are deleted via apoptosis and B-cells via receptor editing and the other is peripheral tolerance, in which the major mechanism appears in regulatory T-cells. While central tolerance causes the loss of autoreactive T-cells during thymus development, peripheral tolerance ensures that autoreactive T-cells that escape central tolerance checkpoints remain unresponsive to pain in peripheral cells [32, 33]. Any defect in an immune tolerance might result in immune dysregulation called autoimmunity, in which the immune response is unable to function properly even when it is not controlled or inhibited. Autoimmune disorders arise when the host immune system damages the normal components of the host body. It can also be defined as the failure to differentiate self from non-self, resulting in the breakage of immune tolerance. Autoimmune disorders are believed to arise due to genetic, epidemiological, and environmental factors. All together, these factors cause a break in self-tolerance of the immune system that ultimately activates the self-reactive lymphocytes via several pathways.

2.3.1 Autoimmune disorders in PIDDs

The molecular mechanisms causing the autoimmune-related immunodeficiency in PIDD patients are multiple but are not completely elucidated. Autoimmunity can occur due to alteration in T-cell central/peripheral tolerance, dysregulation in the differentiation of B-cell differentiation, uncontrolled lymphocyte proliferation, and differentiation, and abnormalities in innate and complement systems, and collectively all these defects contribute to the pathogenic process resulting in autoimmunity [34]. Patients suffering from PIDDs and with the symptoms of autoimmunity influence the quality of life by increasing the medication and higher mortality rate. Autoimmune disorders that occur in PIDDs are classified into two groups—primary immunodeficiency with autoimmune manifestations and primary immunodeficiency with autoimmune diseases having well-defined single-gene defects (**Table 4**) [33].

2.3.1.1 Primary immunodeficiency with autoimmune manifestations

A primary immunodeficiency condition named autoimmune polyglandular syndrome type-1 (APS-1) polyglandular autoimmune (PGA) syndrome type-1, or autoimmune polyendocrinopathy-candidiasis-ectodermal dystrophy (APECED), is characterized by chronic or recurrent Candida yeast infections and autoimmunity

Autoimmune disorders in PIDDs	
Diseases with autoimmune manifestations	**Diseases with well-defined single gene defects**
• Autoimmune polyendocrinopathy, candidiasis, ectodermal dysplasia (APECED or APS-1). • Autoimmune lymphoproliferative syndrome (ALPS). • Immune dysregulation, polyendocrinopathy, enteropathy, and X-linked (IPEX) syndrome	• Common variable immune deficiency (CVID). • Wiskott-Aldrich syndrome (WAS) • Hyper IgE syndrome • STAT5b deficiency • Hyper IgM syndrome. • Idiopathic T-cell lymphopenia (ICL). • Omenn syndrome

Table 4.
Autoimmune disorders in PIDDs.

that affects several endocrine and non-endocrine organs with variable frequency. The majority of APECED patients first exhibit symptoms in early childhood, yet many families find that the interval between symptom start and APECED diagnosis is painfully long. The APECED patients exhibit diverse clinical manifestations, even among affected siblings in the same family, showing that the development of APECED symptoms is influenced by interactions between genetic, epigenetic, and environmental variables. Variants in the autoimmune regulator (AIRE) gene are the main cause of APECED [35, 36]. Autoimmune diseases associated with APECED include hypothyroidism, hypogonadism, type I diabetes, autoimmune hepatitis, pernicious anemia, vitiligo, alopecia, primary biliary cirrhosis, and ectodermal dysplasia. Treatment includes corticosteroids and anti-inflammatory drugs, such as cyclosporine A, and currently, hematopoietic stem cell transplantation is preferred [35].

Autoimmune lymphoproliferative syndrome (ALPS) is a rare hereditary condition in which lymphocytes proliferate and accumulate in the lymph nodes and spleen. It arises due to the dysfunction in the signaling responsible for lymphocyte death. Genetic variations in the FAS gene cause ALPS. It is linked to increases in lymph nodes (lymphadenopathy) and the spleen (splenomegaly) that appear in childhood, which additionally result in a reduction of red blood cells, platelets, and in some cases, neutrophils. Patient suffering from ALPS often have a higher risk of lymphoma. This disease is characterized by lymphadenopathy, splenomegaly, polyclonal hyperimmunoglobulinemia, and autoimmunity. ALPS has many autoimmune manifestations, and autoimmune cytopenias are often severe or worsen with age [37]. Treatment for ALPS depends on the severity of the condition. Short-term steroid treatment of immune cytopenias is usually effective. In severe cases, this includes high doses of the steroid IVIG. Currently, hematopoietic stem cell transplantation is used in severe cases that do not respond to various treatments [38].

Another condition of immune dysregulation is polyendocrinopathy; enteropathy X-linked (IPEX) syndrome is a hereditary immunodeficiency in which patients suffer from severe, early-onset autoimmune disorders due to a defect in the immune system's control and regulation. IPEX is an X-linked in which affected males develop autoimmunity that can affect any organ. The gastrointestinal tract, skin, and endocrine organs, particularly the thyroid gland and pancreas, are the most frequently targeted. As compared to the other immunodeficiencies, in which individuals are prone to frequent or severe infections, infections are not an important concern for most IPEX patients. Rather, autoimmunity develops early in infancy and can be severe. It tends to worsen and spread with age, resulting in a low quality of life and premature death in almost all instances [39]. The treatment for IPEX consists of both supportive care and immune suppression. Hematopoietic stem cell transplantation (HSCT) is the only treatment that has shown improvement for this disease, and it should be considered early [40]. One of the important proteins that is essential for the development and function of regulatory T-cells is FOXP3. Genetic mutations that damage the FOXP3 protein are a primary cause of IPEX [39].

2.3.1.2 Primary immunodeficiency with autoimmune diseases having well-defined single-gene defects

Wiskott-Aldrich syndrome, a rare PIDD characterized by three clinical signs—eczema, a bleeding problem, and increased susceptibility to infections. It is an X-linked disorder caused by a mutation in the WAS gene. The affected individuals have a higher risk of autoimmunity and malignancy. These additional complications in WAS patients result in health challenges that are often not present in other types of PIDD. In some cases, individuals suffer from all three classic signs of WAS, whereas some individuals only suffer from low platelet counts and hemorrhage [41]. Initially, the condition was known as X-linked thrombocytopenia (XLT). It was not until the gene responsible for WAS was found that it became clear that both conditions are caused by mutations in the same gene. XLT patients typically do not have notable immunodeficiency, but they may have a higher risk of autoimmunity and malignancy, but not as WAS.

Omenn syndrome, a PIDD caused by suballelic mutations in RAG1/RAG2 is characterized by expansion of oligoclonal T-cells, increased IgE, erythroderma, lymphadenopathy, and inflammatory bowel disease [42]. Another condition is STAT5b deficiency. It is a rare somatic recessive genetic disease usually associated with mutations in the STAT5b gene. Different variants that cause STAT5b deficiency are associated with different clinical outcomes. Most patients are now treated for growth defects, eczema, lymphocytic interstitial pneumonia, recurrent pneumonia, infections, and autoimmune diseases. Many autoimmune diseases that occur during STAT5b deficiency include autoimmune thrombocytopenia, autoimmune thyroiditis, and rheumatoid arthritis [43]. HyperIgE Syndrome (HIES) is characterized by skin and lung infections and very high IgE levels, mainly caused by *Staphylococcus aureus* and Candida eczema. The autosomal dominant form is caused by dominant-negative heterozygous mutations in the STAT3 gene and is associated with facial features, dental and bone changes, and vascular abnormalities, including aneurysms. Autosomal recessive forms of HIES differ from the autosomal dominant form as they do not have bony or tooth abnormalities and are susceptible to viral diseases and autoimmunity [44]. Hyper-IgM syndromes (HIGMS), a heterogeneous group of disorders caused by abnormalities in Ig class switch recombination (CSR), with or without somatic hypermutation (SHM), result in IgA, IgG, and IgE deficiency and normal or elevated IgM levels. Patients with HIGMS are more likely to suffer from opportunistic infections, develop autoimmunity and autoimmune disorders, and have an increased risk of malignancy. The predominant mutation occurs in the CD40L gene (X-linked HIGMS), followed by mutations in the activation-induced cytidine deaminase (AID) gene, which is critical for CSR and SHM. HIGMS is also linked to gene alterations in UNG, NEMO, and CD40. HIGMS with different gene variants are likely to develop different autoimmune disorders [45].

Immune suppressive medications are used to treat autoimmune conditions, but they may also suppress good and bad autoantibodies and decrease white blood cell types, increasing the risk of infections. Managing these side effects is complex, and a team approach is recommended, involving specialists from various fields, to avoid infections while controlling autoimmune diseases.

3. Conclusion

Clinical immunodeficiency occurs when major immune system components, such as T-cells, B-cells, phagocytes, and complement, are impaired. This can result from intrinsic or heritable defects, failure of normal cellular differentiation, viral infection, or other acquired causes. It increases susceptibility to pathogenic organisms and increases the risk of malignancy, allergy, and autoimmune disease. Immunodeficiency disorders are associated with aberrant immune regulation. Immunocompromised hosts have increased susceptibility to infections due to various factors, including the environment and genetic traits. Understanding these differences can help identify and manage specific pathogens more efficiently.

Conflict of interest

The authors declare no conflict of interest.

Author details

Hajra Fayyaz[1], Atteaya Zaman[1,2], Waheed Rafiq[3], Muhammad Hasnain Murtaza[3] and Imran Ullah[1*]

1 Faculty of Biological Sciences, Department of Biochemistry, Quaid-i-Azam University, Islamabad, Pakistan

2 Department of Biochemistry, Federal Medical and Dental College, Shaheed Zulfiqar Ali Bhutto Medical University, Islamabad, Pakistan

3 Department of Biochemistry, Qauid-i-Azam University, Islamabad, Pakistan

*Address all correspondence to: imranullah@qau.edu.pk

References

[1] McComb S, Thiriot A, Akache B, Krishnan L, Stark F. Introduction to the immune system. In: Immunoproteomics: Methods and Protocols. New York, NY: Humana; 2019. pp. 1-24

[2] Varadé J, Magadán S, González-Fernández Á. Human immunology and immunotherapy: Main achievements and challenges. Cellular & Molecular Immunology. 2021;**18**(4):805-828

[3] Nomula K, Ale H, Chang C. Innate and adaptive immunity. In: Absolute Allergy and Immunology Board Review. Springer International: Cham; 2022. pp. 1-11

[4] Monteleone G, Moscardelli A, Colella A, Marafini I, Salvatori S. Immune-mediated inflammatory diseases: Common and different pathogenic and clinical features. Autoimmunity Reviews. 2023;**22**(10):103410

[5] Ferris MT, Hood DW. Host genetic regulation of immune-based and infectious diseases : Introduction to mammalian genome special issue: Genetics of infectious disease. Mammalian Genome. 2018;**29**(7-8):365-366. DOI: 10.1007/s00335-018-9779-y

[6] Haq IU, Ijaz S, Khan IA. A journey from Koch's postulates to molecular system biology. In: Phytomycology and Molecular Biology of Plant Pathogen Interactions. Boca Raton, USA: CRC Press; 2022. pp. 1-25

[7] Gruenheid S, Skamene E, Gros P. Nramp1: A novel macrophage protein with a key function in resistance to intracellular pathogens. Advances in Cellular and Molecular Biology of Membranes and Organelles. 1999;**5**:345-362

[8] Guo Z, Zhang Z, Prajapati M, Li Y. Lymphopenia caused by virus infections and the mechanisms beyond. Viruses. 2021;**13**(9):1876

[9] Mustafa SS, Rider NL, Jolles S. Immunosuppression in patients with primary immunodeficiency—Walking the line. The Journal of Allergy and Clinical Immunology: In Practice. 2022;**10**(12):3088-3096

[10] Redmond MT, Scherzer R, Prince BT. Novel genetic discoveries in primary immunodeficiency disorders. Clinical Reviews in Allergy & Immunology. 2022;**63**(1):55-74

[11] Lewandowicz-Uszyńska A, Pasternak G, Świerkot J, Bogunia-Kubik K. Primary immunodeficiencies: Diseases of children and adults–a review. Medical and Biomedical Updates. 2021;**1289**:37-54

[12] Abolhassani H, Hammarström L, Cunningham-Rundles C. Current genetic landscape in common variable immune deficiency. Blood, The Journal of the American Society of Hematology. 2020;**135**(9):656-667

[13] Tangye SG, Al-Herz W, Bousfiha A, Cunningham-Rundles C, Franco JL, Holland SM, et al. Human inborn errors of immunity: 2022 update on the classification from the international union of immunological societies expert committee. Journal of Clinical Immunology. 2022;**42**(7):1473-1507

[14] Rispoli F, Valencic E, Girardelli M, Pin A, Tesser A,

Piscianz E, et al. Immunity and genetics at the revolving doors of diagnostics in primary immunodeficiencies. Diagnostics. 2021;**11**(3):532

[15] Kim-Chang JJ, Sleasman JW. Immune deficiencies affecting cellular and humoral immunity T-cell and combined immunodeficiency disorders commonly present in early infancy. If infants present with opportunistic infections such as pneumocystis. Neonatology Questions and Controversies: Infectious Disease, Immunology, and Pharmacology. 2023;**1**:224

[16] Aranda CS, Gouveia-Pereira MP, da Silva CJ, Rizzo MC, Ishizuka E, de Oliveira EB, et al. Severe combined immunodeficiency diagnosis and genetic defects. Immunological Reviews. 2024;**322**(1):138-147

[17] Wadbudhe AM, Meshram RJ, Tidke SC. Severe combined immunodeficiency (SCID) and its new treatment modalities. Cureus. 2023;**15**(10):47759

[18] Dvorak CC, Haddad E, Heimall J, Dunn E, Buckley RH, Kohn DB, et al. The diagnosis of severe combined immunodeficiency (SCID): The primary immune deficiency treatment consortium (PIDTC) 2022 definitions. Journal of Allergy and Clinical Immunology. 2023;**151**(2):539-546

[19] Szczawinska-Poplonyk A, Schwartzmann E, Bukowska-Olech E, Biernat M, Gattner S, Korobacz T, et al. The pediatric common variable immunodeficiency—From genetics to therapy: A review. European Journal of Pediatrics. 2022;**181**:1371-1383

[20] Lee TK, Gereige JD, Maglione PJ. State-of-the-art diagnostic evaluation of common variable immunodeficiency. Annals of Allergy, Asthma & Immunology. 2021;**127**(1):19-27

[21] Alizadeh Z, Dashti P, Mazinani M, Nourizadeh M, Shakerian L, Tajik S, et al. Clinical and genetic study of X-linked agammaglobulinemia patients (the benefit of early diagnosis). Iranian Journal of Allergy, Asthma and Immunology. 2020;**19**(3):305-309

[22] Torralba-Raga LJ. Genetic Predisposition to Immune Cell Malfunction and Inflammation. Sweden: Karolinska Institutet; 2021

[23] Nandiwada SL. Overview of human B-cell development and antibody deficiencies. Journal of Immunological Methods. 2023;**519**:113485

[24] Cirillo E, Giardino G, Grasso F, Gallo V, Pignata C. DiGeorge Syndrome. In: Genetic Syndromes: A Comprehensive Reference Guide. Cham: Springer International Publishing; 2022. pp. 1-7

[25] Obiekwe S, Elhaddad M, Medani K. Thymic transplantation in DiGeorge syndrome. Nigerian Journal of Cardiovascular & Thoracic Surgery. 2021;**6**(2):28-31

[26] Amirifar P, Ranjouri MR, Lavin M, Abolhassani H, Yazdani R, Aghamohammadi A. Ataxia-telangiectasia: Epidemiology, pathogenesis, clinical phenotype, diagnosis, prognosis and management. Expert Review of Clinical Immunology. 2020;**16**(9):859-871

[27] Cinicola BL, Pulvirenti F, Capponi M, Bonetti M, Brindisi G, Gori A, et al. Selective IgA deficiency and allergy: A fresh look to an old story. Medicina. 2022;**58**(1):129

[28] Raj SC, Mahapatra A, Patnaik K, Tabassum S. Neutropenia:

Etiopathogenesis, evaluation and management outcomes. In: Advances in Health and Disease. Nova publications Book; 2021;**36**:69-110

[29] Justiz-Vaillant AA, Williams-Persad AF, Arozarena-Fundora R, Gopaul D, Soodeen S, Asin-Milan O, et al. Chronic granulomatous disease (CGD): Commonly associated pathogens, diagnosis and treatment. Microorganisms. 2023;**11**(9):2233

[30] Morimoto M, Nicoli ER, Kuptanon C, Roney JC, Serra-Vinardell J, Sharma P, et al. Spectrum of LYST mutations in Chediak-Higashi syndrome: A report of novel variants and a comprehensive review of the literature. Journal of Medical Genetics. 2024;**61**(3):212-223

[31] Brodszki N, Frazer-Abel A, Grumach AS, Kirschfink M, Litzman J, Perez E, et al. European society for immunodeficiencies (ESID) and European reference network on rare primary immunodeficiency, autoinflammatory and autoimmune diseases (ERN RITA) complement guideline: Deficiencies, diagnosis, and management. Journal of Clinical Immunology. 2020;**40**:576-591

[32] Goswami TK, Singh M, Dhawan M, Mitra S, Emran TB, Rabaan AA, et al. Regulatory T cells (Tregs) and their therapeutic potential against autoimmune disorders–advances and challenges. Human Vaccines & Immunotherapeutics. 2022;**18**(1):2035117

[33] Gupta S, Louis AG. Tolerance and autoimmunity in primary immunodeficiency disease: A comprehensive review. Clinical Reviews in Allergy & Immunology. 2013;**45**:162-169

[34] Costagliola G, Cappelli S, Consolini R. Autoimmunity in primary immunodeficiency disorders: An updated review on pathogenic and clinical implications. Journal of Clinical Medicine. 2021;**10**(20):4729

[35] Ferré EM, Schmitt MM, Lionakis MS. Autoimmune polyendocrinopathy-candidiasis-ectodermal dystrophy. Frontiers in Pediatrics. 2021;**9**:723532

[36] Kostyuchenko L, Hrytsiuk I, Romanyshyn Y, Bojko Y, Sakovich I. Autoimmune polyendocrinopathy candidiasis ectodermal dystrophy (APECED): Single-Centre experience. Immunology and Genetics Journal. 2021;**4**(1):35-45

[37] Lambert MP. Presentation and diagnosis of autoimmune lymphoproliferative syndrome (ALPS). Expert Review of Clinical Immunology. 2021;**17**(11):1163-1173

[38] Paskiewicz A, Niu J, Chang C. Autoimmune lymphoproliferative syndrome: A disorder of immune dysregulation. Autoimmunity Reviews. 2023;**22**(11):103442

[39] Park JH, Lee KH, Jeon B, Ochs HD, Lee JS, Gee HY, et al. Immune dysregulation, polyendocrinopathy, enteropathy, X-linked (IPEX) syndrome: A systematic review. Autoimmunity Reviews. 2020;**19**(6):102526

[40] Ben-Skowronek I. IPEX syndrome: Genetics and treatment options. Genes. 2021;**12**(3):323

[41] Sudhakar M, Rikhi R, Loganathan SK, Suri D, Singh S. Autoimmunity in Wiskott–Aldrich syndrome: Updated perspectives. The Application of Clinical Genetics. 2021;**14**:363-388

[42] Villa A, Notarangelo LD, Roifman CM. Omenn syndrome:

Inflammation in leaky severe combined immunodeficiency. Journal of Allergy and Clinical Immunology. 2008;**122**(6):1082-1086

[43] Hagin D, STAT5b Deficiency, AR. Encyclopedia of Medical Immunology: Immunodeficiency Diseases. New York, NY: Springer; 2020. pp. 599-609

[44] Gracci S, Novelli T, D'Elios S, Bernardini R, Peroni D. Hyper IgE Syndromes. Current Pediatric Reviews. 2024;**20**(3):253-264

[45] Prakash PR, Gupta G, Adarsh AK, Sashank S, Sinha S. Hyper IgM syndromes: A brief review of the pathogenesis, clinical features and management. Journal of Clinical and Cellular Immunology. 2023;**14**:693

Chapter 2

Innate Immunity in Tuberculosis

Zonghai Chen

Abstract

Tuberculosis (TB) is an airborne infectious disease caused by the *Mycobacterium tuberculosis* (Mtb) complex, which is one of the top 10 causes of death in the world. In recent years, the rising incidence rate of drug-resistant TB has posed a challenge to traditional anti-TB drugs; drug-resistant TB is difficult to treat and seriously threatens public health, so it is urgent to develop new anti-TB drugs. Only 5–10% of infected people will develop tuberculosis post-infection with Mtb, indicating that host innate immunity plays a key role in preventing TB. This chapter discusses the host innate immune defense and immune evasion of Mtb during infection. An in-depth understanding of the mechanisms of pathogen-host interactions can provide an important theoretical basis for the development of new anti-TB drugs.

Keywords: interaction between host and pathogen, immune evasion, innate immune defense, innate immune receptors, *Mycobacterium tuberculosis*, tuberculosis

1. Introduction

In 1882, Robert Koch discovered the pathogen of tuberculosis (TB), the *Mycobacterium tuberculosis* (Mtb) complex, which causes disease through airborne transmission. According to WHO, in 2022, an estimated 10.6 million people developed active TB disease, of whom 1.3 million died [1]. Persistent transmission of Mtb infections and reactivation of latent tuberculosis infections (LTBI) are the causes of TB [2]. The majority of TB is attributed to Mtb or *Mycobacterium africanum*, and a minority of TB is attributed to *Mycobacterium bovis* or *Mycobacterium caprae* [3]. Mtb has no environmental reservoir and humans are its only known reservoir [4]. Mtb is both a pathogen and a commensal, critical to our understanding of host-pathogen interactions.

Mtb is a highly successful intracellular pathogen that has co-evolved with the host over many years. The progression of Mtb infection cannot be separated from its interaction with a variety of host innate immune cells such as macrophages, dendritic cells (DC), neutrophils, and natural killer (NK) cells during the early stages of infection [5]. Host innate immune cells are induced to take on non-sterile control of the Mtb, which leads to latent Mtb infection followed by maintenance of host-pathogen homeostasis through granuloma formation. The reactivation rate of LTBI is 5–10%, suggesting that host innate immunity is critical for the limitation of Mtb infection.

Granulomatous lesions result when host innate immunity is reduced and host cells fail to inhibit the growth of Mtb. Granulomatous lesions induce macrophage death and increase the recruitment of inflammatory cells, exacerbating the disease. The evasion of host immunity by Mtb reflects its strong adaptation in host cells. Host innate immune cells express different pattern recognition receptors (PRRs), such as toll-like receptors (TLRs), c-type lectin receptors (CLRs), and nod-like receptors (NLRs). These receptors not only recognize and uptake Mtb, but also involved in a wide range of innate immunity-associated cellular functions, such as phagocytosis, apoptosis, autophagy, and initiation of inflammasome activation [6–8]. This also limits the development of adaptive immune responses during Mtb infection.

In this chapter, we highlight the process of Mtb infection in the host, the major innate immune cells, PRR-related signaling pathways, and cell function associated with Mtb infection. A better understanding of the molecular mechanisms of host-pathogen interactions can provide an important theoretical basis for developing effective anti-tuberculosis therapies.

2. The process of Mtb infection in the host

Mtb is transmitted in the population by aerosolized particles; the size of infected droplets ranges from 0.65 to 7.0 μm. Small aerosolized particles of Mtb are expected to be deposited in the distal airways *via* the nasopharynx or tracheobronchus, and larger particles may end up in the upper respiratory tract or oropharynx, potentially leading to oropharyngeal or oropharyngeal lymph node tuberculosis [9]. Once Mtb enters the lower respiratory tract, it is mainly phagocytosed by macrophages and DCs. In addition, neutrophils are one of the main phagocytes of Mtb post-infection [10]. Mtb has also been found in non-myeloid granulocytes of TB patients (**Figure 1**) [11]. Mtb that is able to pass through the upper respiratory tract will be delivered to the alveoli. The alveoli are composed of type I and type II epithelial cells and many other immune cells such as alveolar macrophages, DCs, and neutrophils [12]. Mtb can also infect

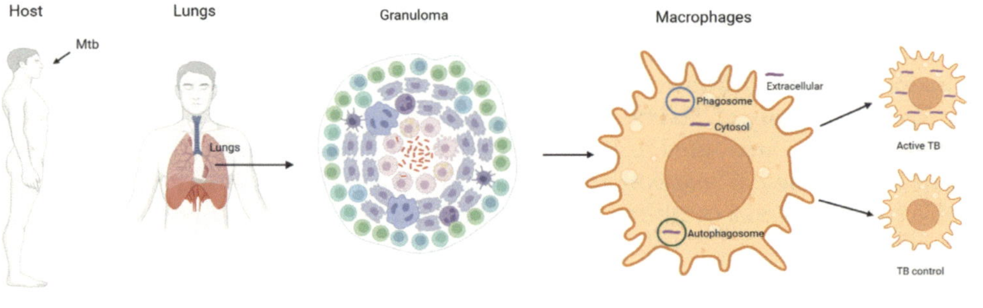

Figure 1.
The process of Mtb infection in the host. Mtb is transmitted in the air as droplet nuclei from an infected person to a susceptible person. Transmission occurs when droplet nuclei of Mtb are inhaled and travel through the oral or nasal cavity, upper respiratory tract, and bronchi to reach the alveoli. Once Mtb colonizes the host, inflammatory cells infiltrate the site of colonization and form characteristic granulomas in the lungs, which are cellular aggregates composed of macrophages, multinucleated giant cells, epithelioid and foam cells, granulocytes, and lymphocytes. Mtb can infect a variety of cell types, primarily macrophages. Once internalized by the cell, Mtb can reside in different cellular compartments such as phagosomes and autophagosomes, and if these organelles are disrupted, Mtb can also enter the cytoplasm. The host will use the innate immune mechanism to control the infection, which will compete with the Mtb immune escape mechanism, and if Mtb succeeds in immune escape, it will be able to survive and replicate in the host.

type II alveolar epithelial cells, and studies have detected Mtb DNA in these cells [13]. Mtb can also invade specialized epithelial microfolded cells in the upper respiratory tract of mice to initiate infection [14]. Infected cells trigger local inflammation to attract immune cells to the site of infection. These cell aggregates form granulomas, a typical pathological feature of tuberculosis. The granuloma structure represents the complex environment of Mtb, which differs greatly from healthy tissue and facilitates bacterial replication and dissemination [15].

In extrapulmonary Mtb can spread to almost any organ, and lymphatic vessels and lymph nodes are the main sites of extrapulmonary TB. In lymph nodes of patients with extrapulmonary TB, Mtb has been found to infect lymphatic endothelial cells (LEC). LEC could provide a niche for Mtb that promotes persistent infection in lymph nodes [16]. In addition, adipose tissue and bone marrow were considered to be extrapulmonary niches where Mtb could survive for long periods [17, 18].

In summary, Mtb can infect different cell types and encounter different environments within these cells. How specific cell type environments affect the localization and survival of Mtb is not known, and these different intracellular environments may have far-reaching consequences in the transmission, progression, and resolution of TB. Among those innate immune cells are critical.

3. Innate immune cells in tuberculosis

The main innate immune cells that play a key role during Mtb infection are macrophages, DCs, neutrophils, and NK cells [19]. In addition, alveolar epithelial cells and endothelial cells have been shown to have an early immune response against Mtb [20]. During Mtb infection, various cells play different but overlapping roles and are susceptible to Mtb regulation. Here, we focus on the regulatory roles of four major types of innate immune cells during Mtb infection.

3.1 Macrophages

Macrophages are critical in Mtb pathogenesis as they are the main cellular niches of Mtb in early and chronic infections. In the lung, macrophages are divided into alveolar macrophages (AM), which are present in the airways, and interstitial macrophages (IM), which are present in the lung parenchyma. AMs maintain airway barrier integrity, lubricate the lung epithelium by regulating the production of surfactant and immunomodulatory cytokines, and also remove dead cells by cell burial. IMs in the lung regulate T cells and DCs by producing IL-10 during infection [21, 22]. Macrophage development and function are driven by microenvironmental signals, of which the M1 and M2 populations are two phenotypes of macrophage polarization. Classically activated M1 macrophages are key effectors of the host response to intracellular bacteria and produce immunostimulatory cytokines that can be induced by LPS, IFNγ, TNFα, and GM-CSF. In contrast, alternatively activated M2 macrophages are poor antigen-presenting cells and suppressors of Th1 responses that can be induced by IL-4 and IL-13 as well as IL-10 and TGFβ [23, 24]. M2-type macrophage plays a crucial role in the promotion and maintenance of Mtb infection.

AMs are critical in the immune response to TB. Mtb is taken up by AMs in the airways, replicates within AMs, and spreads to the lung parenchyma, where Mtb is diffused to other immune cells or stromal cells [25–27]. Immune resistance of AMs can be increased by NRF2-mediated antioxidant pathways early in the infection, but eventually the bacteria disrupt the antimicrobial response of AMs [28]. Mtb manipulates the formation of mature phagosomes in an ESX-1-dependent manner, prolonging their survival within AMs [29]. Mtb infection modulates macrophage autophagy, apoptosis, inflammatory factor production, inflammasome formation, and immune cell crosstalk. Mtb inhibits apoptosis in a host-favorable manner and induces necroptosis by secreting TNF and type I IFN [30, 31]. In particular, macrophage death leads to increased growth and replication of Mtb [32]. Mtb aggregates can avoid phagocytosis by feeding on dead macrophages in an ESX-1- and bacterial lipid dibasic mycobacterial nucleate (PDIM)-dependent manner without requiring live AMs [33]. They go on to kill other macrophages, leading to cell death and inflammation and facilitating the spread of Mtb. AMs infected with Mtb drive the formation of granulomas. Granulomas have been one of the diagnostic indicators of tuberculosis and granulomas lead to disease progression [34, 35]. After Mtb infection, bone marrow-derived monocyte-derived macrophages are recruited to the lungs (IM) within a short period, which are metabolized by glycolysis and have a bacteria-killing capacity. *In vivo* studies in mice revealed a less oxidative stress phenotype and a higher rate of intracellular bacterial replication in AM than IM, suggesting that AM is more susceptible to Mtb. The immune metabolism of these two types of macrophages is also different, with AM having increased fatty acid metabolism and IM relying on glycolysis. Mtb induces an M2-like anti-inflammatory phenotype in AMs, which promotes bacterial replication within these cells, whereas IMs exhibit an M1-like pro-inflammatory phenotype, which limits bacterial replication [36, 37].

In addition to this, Mtb induces the fusion of macrophages to form multinucleated giant cells, which becomes permissive ecological niches for bacterial survival and multiplication [38]. Mtb also initiates the formation of fatty acid-rich foamy macrophages that provide abundant nutrients during Mtb dormancy. These foamy macrophages are characteristic of Mtb granulomas and contain large numbers of replicating bacteria [39]. Human AMs have some antimicrobial capacities, but Mtb induces changes in the macrophage transcriptome, intracellular lipid accumulation, and conversion to an M2 inflammation-suppressing phenotype, thereby disrupting their antimicrobial defenses [40]. *In vivo* studies have shown a similar dependence of Mtb on fatty acid metabolism [41].

Bacillus Calmette-Guerin (BCG) inoculation of mice reprogrammed hematopoietic stem cells in the bone marrow, causing monocyte progenitors to produce more pro-inflammatory macrophages and inhibit virulent Mtb replication. However, myelopoiesis was suppressed in virulent Mtb-inoculated mice, and macrophages failed to control Mtb infection [42, 43]. How Mtb evades the intrinsic immunity of macrophages has not been fully uncovered, and further study of immune escape of Mtb in macrophages, the mechanisms that regulate macrophage polarity, and detailed mechanistic insights into macrophage function in training immunity may contribute to the design of the next-generation Mtb vaccine.

3.2 Dendritic cells

DCs are specialized antigen-presenting cells (APCs) that present peptide antigens *via* endocytosis and load peptide antigens onto MHC-II molecules for subsequent effector with CD4 T cells. Due to antigen presentation, they are an important bridge between intrinsic and adaptive immunities. Mtb is recognized by DCs *via* TLR9 and initiates bacterial uptake [44]. Mtb is processed in the intracellular cytoplasm, and antigens loaded onto MHC-1 are delivered to cytotoxic CD8 T cells to promote their cytokine secretion while recruiting monocytes and neutrophils to kill bacteria [45]. During Mtb infection, both classical and monocyte-derived DCs are important for CD4 T-cell priming. DC-depleted mice have impaired CD4 T-cell responses, induced increased bacterial load, and reduced mouse survival [46]. One study has shown that Mtb antigen drives the activation and proliferation of regulatory T cells in DC-assisted lymph nodes, this delays the activation of effector T cells and retains bacteria in the lungs. In addition, after Mtb infection, the secretion of pro-inflammatory cytokines and integrin levels in dendritic cells is inhibited, leading to a decrease in the adhesion ability of dendritic cells to endothelial cells, which may delay the adaptive T-cell response [47].

Mtb rapidly infects dendritic cells *in vivo* and negatively affects their antigen-presenting function [48, 49]. Mtb prevents DC maturation by inhibiting the release of pro-inflammatory cytokines, and immature DCs are transported inefficiently, rendering the T-cell effector capacity inadequate [50]. Mtb also interferes with the presentation of antigens to dendritic cells. Infected DCs have fewer antigens on MHC-II. The DC subpopulation in the blood of TB patients is depleted from the blood and accumulates in granulomas compared to healthy donors, suggesting that DCs are recruited to the site of disease [51, 52]. Infected DCs in granulomas showed decreased CCR7 expression, suggesting impaired migration and antigen presentation. However, DCs in lymph nodes that could normally induce T-cell responses were not infected by Mtb, suggesting that Mtb limits the innate immune function of DCs and establishes infection [53]. Thus, DCs are a major target of Mtb and crucial to linking host immunity. However, the role of different DC subpopulations and particularly type I IFNs that produce pDCs in TB immunity is unclear. Further understanding of these subpopulations will pave the way for innovative vaccination approaches to prevent Mtb infection.

3.3 Neutrophils

Neutrophils are the most abundant leukocytes in the body and play a crucial role in protective immunity against various pathogens. Neutrophils are the most abundant cell type in bronchoalveolar lavage and sputum from patients with active tuberculosis [54]. Furthermore, neutrophils are the predominant cell type in tissue biopsies of TB patients carrying Mtb [55]. An extensive neutrophilic reaction is a marker of the severity of tuberculosis and is particularly associated with structural lung damage [56].

Neutrophils are the first phagocytes recruited from the vascular system to the interstitium of the lung during tuberculosis. Exposure of humans to Mtb results in neutrophil blood counts that are initially higher than those of unexposed controls. Individuals in contact with TB patients who have high peripheral blood neutrophil counts are less likely to be infected with Mtb. In one study, neutrophils inhibited 50–95% of bacterial growth 1 hour after *in vitro* infection with virulent *Mycobacterium tuberculosis* and TNFα stimulation [57]. Furthermore, neutrophils are early phagocytes in tuberculosis granulomas and kill Mtb by causing oxidative damage [58]. Neutrophil-depleted whole blood has a reduced ability to control Mtb infection *in vitro*. In conclusion, the bactericidal function of neutrophils may be critical for the innate immune control of Mtb.

Tuberculosis lesions in the Mtb highly susceptible strains of mice contained numerous necrotic neutrophils, whereas lesions in the non-susceptible strains of mice contained only a few neutrophils and almost no necrosis. Macrophages phagocytose

Mtb induced necrotic neutrophils and promote bacterial growth. Neutrophil-rich nodule lesions are niches for Mtb, allowing bacterial replication. This suggests that a sustained influx of neutrophils into TB granulomas is responsible for the failure of immune control [59]. In humans, necrotic neutrophils also fail to control Mtb infection [60]. In addition, neutrophil counts in active tuberculosis in humans correlate with poor prognosis [61]. Neutrophils have a dichotomous role in Mtb infection, with an early antibacterial effect and a pro-bacterial survival effect in the chronic phase of infection. Interestingly, neutrophils influence the outcome of granulomas in non-human primates, with neutrophils in granulomas with high bacterial load reducing bacterial replication, whereas neutrophils in granulomas with low load increased the number of bacteria in the granuloma [62]. These results suggest that the extent of neutrophil involvement in pathogenesis varies at the individual granuloma level. Therefore, further study on the role of neutrophils in the post-infection immunity of Mtb, especially their specific functions in different stages of TB, is crucial to clarify the pathogenesis of TB.

3.4 NK cells

NK cells are resident lymphocytes in the lungs that respond rapidly to respiratory infections and are one of the first lines of lung immune defense [63, 64]. NK cells maintain a mature state in the lungs and synthesize and release effector cytokines such as TNFa, IFNg, and GM-CSF in the early stages of infection. NK cells are rapidly recruited into the lungs after infection, releasing effector cytokines and activating cytotoxic T-cell responses [65, 66]. Thus, NK cells are an important bridge between innate and adaptive immunity.

The absence of NK cell activation markers is correlated with active pulmonary tuberculosis [67]. A study showed that the degranulation and IFNg levels of TB patients before treatment were lower than those after treatment [68]. Mtb can be recognized by binding to TLR2 and Nkp44 of NK cells [69]. NK cells then induce cytotoxicity in infected cells, limiting bacterial replication in the early stages of infection [70]. In addition, NK cells regulate effector functions through IFNg and TNFa-mediated formation of reactive oxygen species (ROS) and reactive nitrogen species (RNS) in macrophages and monocytes. IFNg from NK cells is crucial for the survival of Mtb-infected $RAG^{-/-}$ mice [71]. Activation of NK cells post-infection regulates host defense through the rapid accumulation of perforin, granzyme, and IFNg. However, NK cell depletion in C57BL/6 mice showed no alteration in bacterial burden, suggesting that NK cells do not directly regulate TB immunity and that other cells can compensate for NK cell regulation of host defense [72]. Cytokines including IL-2, IL-12, and glutathione can interfere with the outcome of TB by activating NK cell function [73]. NK cells can interact with neutrophils, and NK cells in the lungs inhibit neutrophil inflammation, whereas neutrophil depletion affects NK cell function and activation in Mtb-infected lungs [74]. In addition, NK cells can upregulate the proliferation ability of gd T cells and Mtb-specific CD8+ T cells, promoting Mtb killing. NK cells induce cytotoxicity of iDCs and T-regs, limiting mtb-specific immunity, suggesting that immunomodulatory NK cells play a role in maintaining the balance between adaptive immune effects and regulatory immune effects [75].

NK cells are critical in augmenting the response after vaccination. Long-term NK cell protection was observed in BCG-vaccinated mice, and BCG-vaccinated infants produced significantly more IFNg cells [76]. After Mtb attack, the population of memory NK cells producing IFNg increased in an IL-21-dependent manner,

suggesting that NK cells are important mediators of trained immunity [77].
Most studies of NK cell function in TB have been performed in human peripheral blood or TB-susceptible animal models. However, the role of NK cells in latent TB infection is unclear. Further studies are needed to characterize the exact function of NK cells in all stages of TB disease.

4. Innate immune signaling pathways in tuberculosis

During Mtb infection, the first step in activating innate immunity is to identify pathogens. Multiple conserved PAMPs on the surface of Mtb can be recognized by PRRs on host cells, including TLRs, NLRs, CLRs, CD14 receptors, scavenger receptors, AIM2, and AhR [78, 79]. Innate immune cells recognize Mtb through different receptors or receptor combinations, and Mtb may preferentially act on innate immune cell-specific receptors to suppress immune responses and help their intracellular survival. In addition, a series of studies have shown that protein modification systems play an important role in regulating innate immune signaling pathways [80]. Here, we focus on the regulatory role of the TLR, NLR, and CLR pathways in Mtb infection.

4.1 TLR signaling

TLRs are a type I transmembrane protein family that can recognize the paps and toll interleukin-1 receptor (TIR) domains of pathogens. TLRs can recruit downstream adapters, including MYD88, TRIF, TIRAP, and TRAM. Depending on their cellular localization and agonists, TLRs are classified into two groups: plasma membrane-anchored TLRs (TLR1, 2, 4, 5, and 6) and endosomal TLRs (TLR3, 7, 8, and 9), with plasma membrane-anchored TLRs mainly recognizing microbial membrane components such as LPS, and endosomal TLRs detecting microbial nucleic acids [81]. After pathogen infection, TLRs recruit corresponding adapters to transmit signals downwards and activate signaling pathways such as NF-κB, PI3K/Akt, MAPK, ultimately inducing the release of pro-inflammatory cytokines and/or type I interferons. The activation and expression level of TLRs can reflect the immune status of TB patients. TLR2$^{-/-}$ mice exhibit defective granuloma formation following Mtb infection, and compared to wild-type mice, they have a significantly increased susceptibility to infection. Consistent with the mouse results, TLR2 polymorphisms in humans were associated with enhanced susceptibility to TB [82]. In addition, TLR7 and TLR8 are also closely associated with susceptibility to Mtb infection. Individuals with mutations in TLR7 IVS2-151A and TLR8-129C genes exhibit impaired fusion of phagosomes and lysosomes, leading to insufficient immune levels [83]. The TLR9 knockout mice were also associated with enhanced susceptibility to TB infection. TLR9$^{-/-}$ mice die earlier from Mtb infection than WT mice [84]. However, there is controversy over the protective role of TLRs during Mtb infection. A study revealed that the key factor triggering macrophage effects after Mtb infection is MyD88, not TLRs [85]. Another study showed that pro-inflammatory cytokines can be induced solely by the caspase-1 pathway after Mtb infection, without the involvement of TLRs (**Figure 2**) [86].

Mtb expresses a wide variety of different lipoproteins and lipoglycans that can be recognized by different TLRs. For example, Mtb lpqH can be recognized by TLR2 [87]. Activation of TLR3 by *Mycobacterium* RNA induces IL-10 production in BCG-infected macrophages through the PI3K/AKT signaling pathway. TLR3$^{-/-}$ mice have increased levels of IL-12 and IFN-γ expression and down-regulated levels of IL-10,

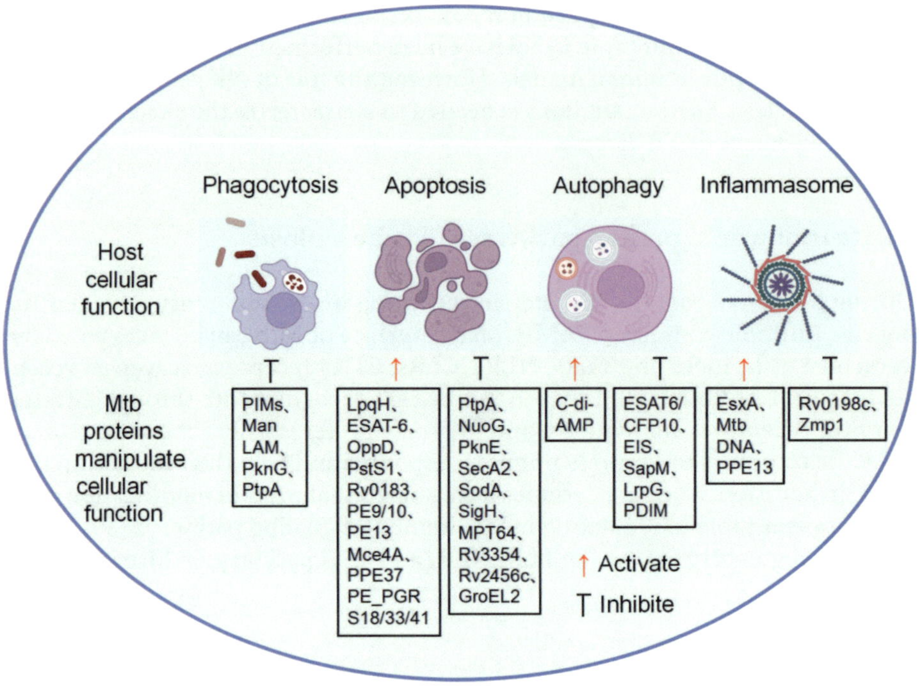

Figure 2.
Mtb components modulate innate immune defense-related cellular functions. During Mtb infection, multiple Mtb components modulate host innate immune defense-related cellular functions such as phagocytosis, apoptotic autophagy, and inflammasome activation to enhance Mtb immune evasion. For example, PIMs, ManLAM, PknG, and PtpA inhibit macrophage phagocytosis by preventing phagocytic vesicle maturation; LpqH, PE_PGRS33, ESAT-6, OppD, PstS1, Rv0183, PE9/PE10, PE13, Mce4A, PPE37, PE_PGRS18, PE_ PGRS33, PE_PGRS41 activate apoptosis, whereas PtpA, NuoG, PknE, SecA2, SodA, SigH, MPT64, Rv3354, Rv2456c, and GroEL2 inhibit apoptosis; C-di-AMP activates autophagy, whereas ESAT6/CFP10, EIS, SapM, LrpG, and PDIM inhibited autophagy; EsxA, Mtb DNA and PPE13 activated inflammasome, while Rv0198c and Zmp1 inhibited inflammasome activation.

which results in a reduction of bacterial burden and tissue damage [88]. Mtb rLrp is activated through the tlr2-mediated activation of the PI3K/AKT pathway, which inhibits the production of pro-inflammatory cytokines and downregulates macrophage antigen presentation [89]. PPE60 drives the Th1/Th17 response by inducing TLR2-dependent DCs maturation and has the potential to be used as an immune vaccine for Mtb [90]. Mtb-secreted proteins such as PtpA and Mce3E have a potential for immunological vaccination by targeting molecules involved in the NF-κB and MAPK pathways to regulate the TLR signaling pathway [91, 92]. In addition, activation of CD40 and TLR4 promotes the release of IL-12, IL-6, and TNF-α from DC cells and limiting Mtb replication [93]. The TLR signaling pathway plays a key role in TB development, and further studies are needed to investigate the potential mechanisms underlying the interactions between the TLR signaling pathway and Mtb components.

4.2 NLR signaling

Members of the NLR family, including NOD1, NOD2, NLRP3, and NLRC4, are intracellular proteins involved in microbial component recognition and activation of inflammatory pathways that protect against pathogen invasion. Mtb is able to escape from the phagolysosome into the cytoplasm of the macrophage by a pathway that is dependent on ESX-1 [94]. Thus, cytoplasmic PRRs such as NOD1 and NOD2 regulate the innate immunity of Mtb. A study in NOD2$^{-/-}$ mice has confirmed the role of NOD2 in Mtb immune defense. Furthermore, in Mtb-infected human alveolar macrophages, activation of NOD2 by cytosolic dipeptides increased cellular control of bacterial growth and recruited autophagy-associated proteins to bacterial-containing autophagic vesicles, highlighting the possibility of PRR-dependent autophagy-activating mechanisms [95]. In addition, a study of African Americans in the United States demonstrated that three common non-synonymous polymorphisms in the NOD2 gene are associated with TB genetic susceptibility [96]. In addition, NLRP3 also plays an important role in Mtb infection. ESAT-6 activates NLRP3/ASC inflammasomes in macrophages, leading to the release of IL-1 β and cell pyroptosis [29]. In addition, PPE13 is involved in the assembly of NLRP3 inflammasome [97]. EST12 can activate NLRP3 *via* the RACK1 to activate NLRP3 [98]. Mtb infection upregulates MFN2 expression to promote NLRP3 inflammasome formation [99]. Thus, Mtb may trigger the activation of inflammasome to promote persistent infection rather than acting as a virulence mechanism. However, PE12 binds to the TLR4 receptor and inhibits NLRP3 activity and inflammatory responses, promoting intracellular survival of Mtb [100]. PknF downregulates NLRP3 activity and promotes intracellular survival of Mtb. Infection by PknF-deficient Mtb strains is associated with an up-regulation of NLRP3 activity, and cellular scorch death occurs in BMDM [101]. Although there are many challenges in the discovery of new NLRs, their role in host rapid progresses in defense against Mtb infection. However, much remains to be learned about the NLR-induced signaling pathways. Elucidating the regulatory functions and mechanisms controlling NLR signaling during Mtb infection is crucial for targeted control of TB.

4.3 CLR signaling

CLR receptors include collecting proteins, phagocytic receptors, selectins, and proteoglycans. Multiple CLRs are associated with Mtb immune response, such as Mr, DCSIGN, Dectin-1/2/3, Mincle, CL-LK, and DCIR. And ligands of Mtb, such as ManLAM and spinal factors, can be directly recognized by CLRs [102, 103]. One study demonstrated the anti-inflammatory effects of DC-SIGN in human IL-4-activated macrophage responses to Mtb [104]. Dectin-1 cooperates with TLR2 to activate pro-inflammatory macrophage responses during mycobacterial infection [105]. Dectin-2 contributes to host immunity to *Mycobacterium* infection by acting as a direct receptor for Mtb ManLAM [106]. The direct binding of Dectin-2 to ManLAM regulates host immunity after mycobacterial infection [107]. A study found that Dectin-3 upregulates the expression of Mincle and promotes Mincle-mediated signal transduction [108]. In addition, the set element CL-LK can recognize and combine with ManLAM [109]. Dectin-2 is involved in regulating the level of type I interferon in DCs and intervening in the immune response after Mtb infection. However, the Mtb ligand of DCIR is not clear [110]. Further understanding of the recognition mechanism of CLRs toward Mtb and the interaction between CLRs and other PRRs on immune cells are of great significance for a more comprehensive understanding of the host innate immune mechanism after Mtb infection.

5. Defense-related cellular functions of innate immune cells in tuberculosis

The recognition of Mtb by innate immune cells triggers various cellular events, such as phagocytosis, autophagy, apoptosis, and inflammasome activation, to restrict or clear Mtb, enhance cell antigen presentation ability, and induce adaptive immunity [110]. In addition, other cellular functions such as the generation of intracellular reactive oxygen species, reactive nitrogen species, antigen presentation, and MHC-II class transport also play important roles in Mtb infection [111]. Here, we focus on the regulation of cellular phagocytosis, apoptosis, autophagy, and inflammasome activation during Mtb infection.

5.1 Phagocytosis

Mtb invades the host innate immune cells through phagocytosis and then holds and replicates in the infected cell by preventing phagosome maturation. This mechanism allows pathogens to avoid contact with acidic environments, lysosomal hydrolases, and bactericidal lysosomal components. Multiple Mtb factors inhibit the maturation of phagosomes. Mtb pim inhibits phagosomal acidification by facilitating phagosome-early nuclear endosome fusion [112]. PIMs may act on Rab14, a GTPase, promoting phagocytic early endosome fusion and inhibiting phagocytic acidification [113]. Mtb ManLAM can bind to MR to limit the maturation of phagosomes [114]. Mtb PknG also has the ability to inhibit the fusion of phagosomes and lysosomes [115]. A study found that Mtb PtpA can inhibit vacuolar acidification by binding to the H subunit of macrophage vacuolar H^+-ATPase [116]. In addition, an acidic and phagocytic vesicle regulatory site (aprABC) was found to respond to acidic stress and regulate the synthesis and segregation of cell wall lipids in strongly toxic Mtb, thereby allowing Mtb to survive under low pH conditions [117]. The antiviral interferon-induced transmembrane protein (IFITM) restricts the survival of mycobacteria in macrophages by inducing the maturation of phagosomes. IFITM3 can interact with V-ATPase and may stabilize its association with the phagosome membrane [118]. However, the mechanism by which Mtb inhibits phagosome maturation remains incompletely understood and requires further study.

5.2 Apoptosis

Apoptosis is an important defense mechanism of the host against pathogens, involving multiple components and complex signaling pathways. Apoptosis is a highly regulated and controlled process, and the two explicit mechanisms of activation of apoptosis are the extrinsic and intrinsic pathways. The external pathway is initiated by the binding of extracellular ligands to cell surface death receptors, leading to the formation of death inducing signaling complexes. The intrinsic pathway is activated by intracellular signals and depends on mitochondria [119]. Apoptosis can induce an acquired cellular immune response in addition to limiting the growth of Mtb during the early stages of infection [120]. Blocking cell apoptosis may be one of the ways in which Mtb immune escape occurs. Mtb has evolved multiple effective mechanisms to manipulate the apoptosis of innate immune cells, and numerous Mtb effector factors are closely related to apoptosis. Known anti-apoptotic Mtb antigens include GroEL2, MPT64, NuoG, PtpA, PknE, Rv3354, Rv2456c, SecA2, SodA, SigH [121–130]. Known pro-apoptotic Mtb antigens include ESAT-6, LpqH, Mce4A, OppD, PE_PGRS33,

PstS1, PE9/PE10, PPE37, PE_PGRS41, PE13, PE_PGRS18, Rv0183 [131–143]. TLRs are also involved in triggering apoptosis in mtb-infected cells. Mtb PE_PGRS33 induces macrophage apoptosis through TLR2 [144]. The PE/PPE complex PE9/PE10 induces macrophage apoptosis through the involvement of TLR4 [137]. Accurately regulating the apoptosis of innate immune cells is an critical strategy for the immune escape of Mtb. Clarifying the regulation mechanism of host innate immune cell apoptosis during infection is conducive to the development of new treatment methods for tuberculosis.

5.3 Autophagy

Autophagy is an inducible intracellular process by which cells eliminate intracellular pathogens, protein aggregates, and damaged organelles. Autophagy begins with the formation of double-membrane-enclosed autophagic follicles [145]. Nutritional deficiencies or IFN-γ treatment induces autophagy in Mtb-infected cells, and bacterial-containing phagosomes acquire lysosomal markers and are acidified [146].

Mtb replicates in macrophages in part by inhibiting phagosome-lysosome fusion until IFN-c activates macrophages to transport Mtb to lysosomes [147]. The role of autophagy in Mtb infection was mainly obtained through macrophage or DC-related studies, in which Mtb was co-localized with autophagy-associated proteins such as ATG5, ATG12, ATG16L1, p62, NDP52, CALCOCO2, and LC3 [148–151]. Induction of autophagy enhances intracellular bacterial killing and inhibition of autophagy increases intracellular bacterial survival [152, 153]. During Mtb infection, of all ATG genes, Mtb persistence was significantly altered only in monocyte-derived cells and neutrophils derived from $ATG5^{-/-}$ mice [154]. In addition, ATG5 is critical in autophagic vesicle formation, and $ATG5^{-/-}$ mice show an increased Mtb burden and die from infection 30 days post-infection [155].

Autophagy protects the host by activating the antimicrobial response of infected cells. LPS treatment induces macrophage autophagy *via* tlr4 to limit Mtb intracellular survival [156]. Immune-related GTPase family M (IRGM) also induces macrophage autophagy to limit Mtb intracellular survival [157]. In addition, the IRGM gene variant between active TB and latent TB infection (LTBI) differs, suggesting that the IRGM genotype may determine whether progression from LTBI to active TB disease occurs [158, 159]. Cyclic di-adenosine monophosphate (C-di-AMP) can also drive type I IFN responses and autophagy in Mtb-infected hosts [160]. Mtb can utilize Rab GTPases to inhibit autophagy, making innate immune cells the replication niche of Mtb. Rab5 is recruited in the early stages of phagosomes containing Mtb, and Mtb inhibits lysosome-phagosome fusion by selectively excluding Rab7 and lysosome-associated membrane protein-1 (LAMP1) [161]. Rab22a, on the other hand, prevents the acquisition of Rab7 and inhibits entry into the late endosomal/lysosomal compartment of the mature endosome [162]. In addition, it has been found that Rab10 is acquired long before acquired before Rab5 and regulates the maturation of mtb-containing phagosomes upstream [163]. Mtb-secreted proteins can inhibit the maturation of phagosomes. ESAT-6/CFP10 regulates the expression of autophagy related genes, inhibits autophagosome maturation, and reduces Mtb clearance [164]. Eis can inhibit phagosome maturation and reactive oxygen species production through direct acetylation of c-Jun-terminal kinase (JNK)-specific phosphatases, enhancing Mtb intracellular survival [165]. SapM inhibits phagosome maturation and promotes pathogen growth in guinea pigs [166]. LrpG blocks phagosome-lysosome fusion in macrophages through a traffic mechanism [167]. PDIM was shown to promote the phagosomal escape of Mtb [168]. In conclusion, despite our growing understanding of the regulatory role of autophagy during Mtb infection, how different Mtb effector proteins synergistically regulate host autophagy in favor of Mtb infection has not been fully explored. Further studies of autophagy in innate immune cells after Mtb infection may open new avenues for the development of new anti-TB drugs.

5.4 Inflammasome activation

During microbial infection, NLRP3 and NLRC4 of the NLR family assemble with the cytoplasmic DNA sensor AIM2 to form a poly inflammasome complex that mediates activation of caspase-1. Subsequently, it leads to the maturation of pro-inflammatory cytokines and induces pyroptosis, a form of necrosis and inflammatory programmed cell death induced by inflammatory cysteine asparaginase [169]. Inflammasomes containing the Pyrin structural domain, including NLRP3 and AIM2, signal through the adapter protein ASC to recruit caspase-1. In contrast, the CARD structural domain-containing inflammasome NLRC4 can signal directly to caspase-1, which leads to focal death, and also indirectly through ASC to increase the secretion of IL-1β and IL-18 [170].

Mtb infection induced an increase in K^+ and Cl^- efflux but had no effect on Ca^{2+} flux. Phagosomal and mitochondrial ROS are not involved in the activation of NLRP3 inflammasome, but rather cytoplasmic ROS is produced by xanthine oxidase In Mtb infection [101]. Interestingly, ESX-1 system-mediated plasma membrane damage triggers an increase in K^+ efflux, which activates NLRP3 inflammasome and pyroptosis, thereby permitting the spread of Mtb to neighboring cells [171]. The AIM2 inflammasome also participates in the recognition of Mtb macrophages, and AIM2 directly binds to the genomic DNA of *Mycobacterium* [78]. Mtb-secreted protein can regulate inflammasome response. Rv0198c can inhibit caspase-1 activation and IL-1β secretion. Zmp1-deficient Mtb triggers the activation of inflammasomes and the release of IL-1 β, promoting the intracellular clearance of Mtb [172]. PPE13 is involved in the assembly of the NLRP3 inflammatory vesicle complex [97]. EST12 binds to the activated C kinase 1 (RACK1) receptor and forms the EST12-RACK1 complex in macrophages, inducing NLRP3 deubiquitination and triggering NLRP3 inflammasome-mediated cell pyroptosis and IL-1β secretion [98]. To further explore the mechanism of inflammasome activation and regulation of innate immune cells after Mtb infection can provide a new direction for anti-TB treatment.

6. Innate immune response in multidrug-resistant tuberculosis

Multidrug-resistant tuberculosis (MDR-TB) is a disease caused by isoniazid and rifampicin-resistant Mtb infection. In recent years, the incidence rate and mortality of MDR-TB cases have remained high, which is a major threat to global public health security [1]. A study of macaques *in vivo* showed that compared with the Mtb strain that is sensitive to drug treatment, the bacterial counts in the airway were higher after MDR-TB infection [173]. This reveals a stronger retention ability *in vivo* caused by MDR Mtb.

MDR Mtb infection induces metabolic changes in macrophages, showing a shift toward aerobic glycolysis and a tendency toward M1 polarity [174]. A study has shown that the cell wall lipids of MDR-TB strains are modified with PDIM, and overexpression of PDIM can directly activate IFN β response, thereby inducing a shift in macrophage metabolism toward aerobic glycolysis and tending toward M1 polarity [175]. However, macrophages in MDR-TB patients tend to be M2 polarity [176]. A study has found that the levels of IL-10, IFNg, and TNF-a in the plasma of MDR-TB patients are elevated, which also supports M2 polarity [177]. This suggests that early induction of M1 type macrophages after MDR Mtb infection, and long-term retention in the human body, leads to M2 polarity of macrophages. A study found that compared to normal peripheral blood neutrophils, MDR strain infection caused a decrease in neutrophil oxidative burst capacity, attributed to decreased phagocytic ability and reduced lipid raft formation [178]. MDR Mtb can inhibit cell apoptosis in both macrophages and neutrophils, thus remaining in the cell [179]. Inducing innate immune cell apoptosis may be a valuable new approach for MDR-TB therapy.

7. Conclusion

Host innate immune cells, PRRs signaling pathways, and immune defense-related cellular functions are critical for limiting TB disease. Innate immune cells play a key role in maintaining the balance between protective and pathogenic immune responses in TB, leading to disease when pathogenic immune responses exceed protective responses. However, Mtb can evade the immune response to antimicrobial drugs and disrupt the dialog between intrinsic and adaptive immunity, thereby skewing the balance toward pathogenic consequences. A series of studies have clearly shown that Mtb manipulates host innate immunity by inducing a complex program involving multiple host signaling pathways and cellular functions. With the increasing incidence of drug-resistant tuberculosis, Mtb infection remains a global public health problem, and clarifying the pathogen-host relationship during Mtb infection will provide theoretical support for the development of new anti-TB drugs.

Acknowledgements

I thank members of Taizhou University Medical School for helpful discussions. I would like to acknowledge the funding of the Science and Technology Projects of Taizhou (24ywb110).

Conflict of interest

The authors declare no conflict of interest.

Author details

Zonghai Chen
Taizhou University Medical School, Taizhou, China

*Address all correspondence to: zonghaichen@163.com

References

[1] Bagcchi S. WHO's global tuberculosis report 2022. The Lancet Microbe. 2023;**4**:e20. DOI: 10.1016/S2666-5247(22)00359-7

[2] Pai M, Behr MA, Dowdy D, Dheda K, Divangahi M, Boehme CC, et al. Tuberculosis. Nature Reviews Disease Primers. 2016;**2**:16076. DOI: 10.1038/nrdp.2016.76

[3] Bos KI, Harkins KM, Herbig A, Coscolla M, Weber N, Comas I, et al. Pre-Columbian mycobacterial genomes reveal seals as a source of New World human tuberculosis. Nature. 2014;**514**:494-497. DOI: 10.1038/nature13591

[4] Comas I, Coscolla M, Luo T, Borrell S, Holt KE, Kato-Maeda M, et al. Out-of-Africa migration and Neolithic co-expansion of *Mycobacterium tuberculosis* with modern humans. Nature Genetics. 2013;**45**:1176-1182. DOI: 10.1038/ng.2744

[5] Chai Q, Lu Z, Liu CH. Host defense mechanisms against *Mycobacterium tuberculosis*. Cellular and Molecular Life Sciences: CMLS. 2020;**77**:1859-1878. DOI: 10.1007/s00018-019-03353-5

[6] Killick KE, Ni CC, O'Farrelly C, Hokamp K, MacHugh DE, Harris J. Receptor-mediated recognition of mycobacterial pathogens. Cellular Microbiology. 2013;**15**:1484-1495. DOI: 10.1111/cmi.12161

[7] Zihad S, Sifat N, Islam MA, Monjur-Al-Hossain A, Sikdar K, Sarker M, et al. Role of pattern recognition receptors in sensing *Mycobacterium tuberculosis*. Heliyon. 2023;**9**:e20636. DOI: 10.1016/j.heliyon.2023.e20636

[8] Khan N, Vidyarthi A, Javed S, Agrewala JN. Innate immunity holding the flanks until reinforced by adaptive immunity against *Mycobacterium tuberculosis* infection. Frontiers in Microbiology. 2016;**7**:328. DOI: 10.3389/fmicb.2016.00328

[9] Fennelly KP, Jones-López EC. Quantity and quality of inhaled dose predicts immunopathology in tuberculosis. Frontiers in Immunology. 2015;**6**:313. DOI: 10.3389/fimmu.2015.00313

[10] Borkute RR, Woelke S, Pei G, Dorhoi A. Neutrophils in tuberculosis: Cell biology, cellular networking and multitasking in host defense. International Journal of Molecular Sciences. 2021;**22**:4801. DOI: 10.3390/ijms22094801

[11] Lerner TR, Borel S, Gutierrez MG. The innate immune response in human tuberculosis: Innate immune response in tuberculosis. Cellular Microbiology. 2015;**17**:1277-1285. DOI: 10.1111/cmi.12480

[12] Ganbat D, Seehase S, Richter E, Vollmer E, Reiling N, Fellenberg K, et al. Mycobacteria infect different cell types in the human lung and cause species dependent cellular changes in infected cells. BMC Pulmonary Medicine. 2016;**16**:19. DOI: 10.1186/s12890-016-0185-5

[13] Hernandez-Pando R, Jeyanathan M, Mengistu G, Aguilar D, Orozco H, Harboe M, et al. Persistence of DNA from *Mycobacterium tuberculosis* in superficially normal lung tissue during latent infection. Lancet. 2000;**356**:2133-2138. DOI: 10.1016/s0140-6736(00)03493-0

[14] Nair VR, Franco LH, Zacharia VM, Khan HS, Stamm CE, You W, et al. Microfold cells actively translocate *Mycobacterium tuberculosis* to initiate infection. Cell Reports (Cambridge). 2016;**16**:1253-1258. DOI: 10.1016/j.celrep.2016.06.080

[15] Rubin EJ. The granuloma in tuberculosis—Friend or foe? The New England Journal of Medicine. 2009;**360**:2471-2473. DOI: 10.1056/NEJMcibr0902539

[16] Lerner TR, Borel S, Greenwood DJ, Repnik U, Russell MRG, Herbst S, et al. Mycobacterium tuberculosis replicates within necrotic human macrophages. Journal of Cell Biology. 2017;**216**:583-594. DOI: 10.1083/jcb.201603040

[17] Beigier-Bompadre M, Montagna GN, Kühl AA, Lozza L, Weiner RJ, Kupz A, et al. Mycobacterium tuberculosis infection modulates adipose tissue biology. PLoS Pathogens. 2017;**13**:e1006676. DOI: 10.1371/journal.ppat.1006676

[18] Mayito J, Andia I, Belay M, Jolliffe DA, Kateete DP, Reece ST, et al. Anatomic and cellular niches for *Mycobacterium tuberculosis* in latent tuberculosis infection. The Journal of Infectious Diseases. 2019;**219**:685-694. DOI: 10.1093/infdis/jiy579

[19] Gold MC, Napier RJ, Lewinsohn DM. MR1-restricted mucosal associated invariant T (MAIT) cells in the immune response to *Mycobacterium tuberculosis*. Immunological Reviews. 2015;**264**:154-166. DOI: 10.1111/imr.12271

[20] Van Rhijn I, Moody DB. CD1 and mycobacterial lipids activate human T cells. Immunological Reviews. 2015;**264**:138-153. DOI: 10.1111/imr.12253

[21] Bain CC, MacDonald AS. The impact of the lung environment on macrophage development, activation and function: Diversity in the face of adversity. Mucosal Immunology. 2022;**15**:223-234. DOI: 10.1038/s41385-021-00480-w

[22] Aegerter H, Lambrecht BN, Jakubzick CV. Biology of lung macrophages in health and disease. Immunity (Cambridge, Mass.). 2022;**55**:1564-1580. DOI: 10.1016/j.immuni.2022.08.010

[23] Murray PJ. Macrophage polarization. Annual Review of Physiology. 2017;**79**:541-566. DOI: 10.1146/annurev-physiol-022516-034339

[24] Ginhoux F, Schultze JL, Murray PJ, Ochando J, Biswas SK. New insights into the multidimensional concept of macrophage ontogeny, activation and function. Nature Immunology. 2016;**17**:34-40. DOI: 10.1038/ni.3324

[25] Upadhyay S, Mittal E, Philips JA. Tuberculosis and the art of macrophage manipulation. Pathogens and Disease. 22018;**76**:fty037. DOI: 10.1093/femspd/fty037

[26] Cohen SB, Gern BH, Delahaye JL, Adams KN, Plumlee CR, Winkler JK, et al. Alveolar macrophages provide an early *Mycobacterium tuberculosis* niche and initiate dissemination. Cell Host & Microbe. 2018;**24**:439-446. DOI: 10.1016/j.chom.2018.08.001

[27] Pisu D, Huang L, Narang V, Theriault M, Le-Bury G, Lee B, et al. Single cell analysis of *M. tuberculosis* phenotype and macrophage lineages in the infected lung. The Journal of Experimental Medicine. 2021;**218**:e20210615. DOI: 10.1084/jem.20210615

[28] Rothchild AC, Olson GS, Nemeth J, Amon LM, Mai D,

Gold ES, et al. Alveolar macrophages generate a noncanonical NRF2-driven transcriptional response to *Mycobacterium tuberculosis* in vivo. Science Immunology. 2019;**4**:eaaw6693. DOI: 10.1126/sciimmunol.aaw6693

[29] Mishra BB, Moura-Alves P, Sonawane A, Hacohen N, Griffiths G, Moita LF, et al. *Mycobacterium tuberculosis* protein ESAT-6 is a potent activator of the NLRP3/ASC inflammasome. Cellular Microbiology. 2010;**12**:1046-1063. DOI: 10.1111/j.1462-5822.2010.01450.x

[30] Pajuelo D, Gonzalez-Juarbe N, Tak U, Sun J, Orihuela CJ, Niederweis M. NAD(+) depletion triggers macrophage necroptosis, a cell death pathway exploited by *Mycobacterium tuberculosis*. Cell Reports. 2018;**24**:429-440. DOI: 10.1016/j.celrep.2018.06.042

[31] Behar SM, Remold HG, Divangahi M. Evasion of innate immunity by *Mycobacterium tuberculosis*: Is death an exit strategy? Nature Reviews. Microbiology. 2010;**8**:668-674. DOI: 10.1038/nrmicro2387

[32] Mahamed D, Boulle M, Ganga Y, Mc AC, Skroch S, Oom L, et al. Intracellular growth of *Mycobacterium tuberculosis* after macrophage cell death leads to serial killing of host cells. eLife. 2017;**6**:e22028. DOI: 10.7554/eLife.22028

[33] Toniolo C, Dhar N, McKinney JD. Uptake-independent killing of macrophages by extracellular *Mycobacterium tuberculosis* aggregates. The EMBO Journal. 2023;**42**:e113490. DOI: 10.15252/embj.2023113490

[34] Pagan AJ, Ramakrishnan L. Immunity and immunopathology in the tuberculous granuloma. Cold Spring Harbor Perspectives in Medicine. 2014;**5**:a018499. DOI: 10.1101/cshperspect.a018499

[35] Marakalala MJ, Raju RM, Sharma K, Zhang YJ, Eugenin EA, Prideaux B, et al. Inflammatory signaling in human tuberculosis granulomas is spatially organized. Nature Medicine. 2016;**22**:531-538. DOI: 10.1038/nm.4073

[36] Ahmad F, Rani A, Alam A, Zarin S, Pandey S, Singh H, et al. Macrophage: A cell with many faces and functions in tuberculosis. Frontiers in Immunology. 2022;**13**:747799. DOI: 10.3389/fimmu.2022.747799

[37] Zhang Y, Li S, Liu Q, Long R, Feng J, Qin H, et al. *Mycobacterium tuberculosis* heat-shock protein 16.3 induces macrophage M2 polarization through CCRL2/CX3CR1. Inflammation. 2020;**43**:487-506. DOI: 10.1007/s10753-019-01132-9

[38] Guirado E, Schlesinger LS, Kaplan G. Macrophages in tuberculosis: Friend or foe. Seminars in Immunopathology. 2013;**35**:563-583. DOI: 10.1007/s00281-013-0388-2

[39] Laval T, Chaumont L, Demangel C. Not too fat to fight: The emerging role of macrophage fatty acid metabolism in immunity to *Mycobacterium tuberculosis*. Immunological Reviews. 2021;**301**:84-97. DOI: 10.1111/imr.12952

[40] Lavalett L, Rodriguez H, Ortega H, Sadee W, Schlesinger LS, Barrera LF. Alveolar macrophages from tuberculosis patients display an altered inflammatory gene expression profile. Tuberculosis (Edinburgh, Scotland). 2017;**107**:156-167. DOI: 10.1016/j.tube.2017.08.012

[41] Chandra P, He L, Zimmerman M, Yang G, Koster S, Ouimet M, et al. Inhibition of fatty acid oxidation promotes macrophage control of

Mycobacterium tuberculosis. MBio. 2020;**11**:e01139-20. DOI: 10.1128/mBio.01139-20

[42] Kaufmann E, Sanz J, Dunn JL, Khan N, Mendonca LE, Pacis A, et al. BCG educates hematopoietic stem cells to generate protective innate immunity against tuberculosis. Cell. 2018;**172**:176-190. DOI: 10.1016/j.cell.2017.12.031

[43] Khan N, Downey J, Sanz J, Kaufmann E, Blankenhaus B, Pacis A, et al. *M. tuberculosis* reprograms hematopoietic stem cells to limit myelopoiesis and impair trained immunity. Cell. 2020;**183**:752-770. DOI: 10.1016/j.cell.2020.09.062

[44] Guilliams M, Lambrecht BN, Hammad H. Division of labor between lung dendritic cells and macrophages in the defense against pulmonary infections. Mucosal Immunology. 2013;**6**:464-473. DOI: 10.1038/mi.2013.14

[45] Khan N, Vidyarthi A, Pahari S, Agrewala JN. Distinct strategies employed by dendritic cells and macrophages in restricting *Mycobacterium tuberculosis* infection: Different philosophies but same desire. International Reviews of Immunology. 2016;**35**:386-398. DOI: 10.3109/08830185.2015.1015718

[46] Tian T, Woodworth J, Skold M, Behar SM. In vivo depletion of CD11c+ cells delays the CD4+ T cell response to *Mycobacterium tuberculosis* and exacerbates the outcome of infection. Journal of Immunology. 2005;**175**:3268-3272. DOI: 10.4049/jimmunol.175.5.3268

[47] Roberts LL, Robinson CM. *Mycobacterium tuberculosis* infection of human dendritic cells decreases integrin expression, adhesion and migration to chemokines. Immunology. 2014;**141**:39-51. DOI: 10.1111/imm.12164

[48] Wolf AJ, Linas B, Trevejo-Nunez GJ, Kincaid E, Tamura T, Takatsu K, et al. *Mycobacterium tuberculosis* infects dendritic cells with high frequency and impairs their function in vivo. Journal of Immunology. 2007;**179**:2509-2519. DOI: 10.4049/jimmunol.179.4.2509

[49] Madan-Lala R, Sia JK, King R, Adekambi T, Monin L, Khader SA, et al. *Mycobacterium tuberculosis* impairs dendritic cell functions through the serine hydrolase Hip1. The Journal of Immunology. 1950;**2014**(192):4263-4272. DOI: 10.4049/jimmunol.1303185

[50] Georgieva M, Sia JK, Bizzell E, Madan-Lala R, Rengarajan J. *Mycobacterium tuberculosis* GroEL2 modulates dendritic cell responses. Infection and Immunity. 2018;**86**:e00387-17. DOI: 10.1128/IAI.00387-17

[51] Uehira K, Amakawa R, Ito T, Tajima K, Naitoh S, Ozaki Y, et al. Dendritic cells are decreased in blood and accumulated in granuloma in tuberculosis. Clinical Immunology. 2002;**105**:296-303. DOI: 10.1006/clim.2002.5287

[52] Lichtner M, Rossi R, Mengoni F, Vignoli S, Colacchia B, Massetti AP, et al. Circulating dendritic cells and interferon-alpha production in patients with tuberculosis: Correlation with clinical outcome and treatment response. Clinical and Experimental Immunology. 2006;**143**:329-337. DOI: 10.1111/j.1365-2249.2005.02994.x

[53] Harding JS, Rayasam A, Schreiber HA, Fabry Z, Sandor M. Mycobacterium-infected dendritic cells disseminate granulomatous inflammation. Scientific Reports. 2015;**5**:15248. DOI: 10.1038/srep15248

[54] Muefong CN, Sutherland JS. Neutrophils in tuberculosis-associated

inflammation and lung pathology. Frontiers in Immunology. 2020;**11**:962. DOI: 10.3389/fimmu.2020.00962

[55] Eum SY, Kong JH, Hong MS, Lee YJ, Kim JH, Hwang SH, et al. Neutrophils are the predominant infected phagocytic cells in the airways of patients with active pulmonary TB. Chest. 2010;**137**:122-128. DOI: 10.1378/chest.09-0903

[56] Sutherland JS, Jeffries DJ, Donkor S, Walther B, Hill PC, Adetifa IM, et al. High granulocyte/lymphocyte ratio and paucity of NKT cells defines TB disease in a TB-endemic setting. Tuberculosis (Edinburgh, Scotland). 2009;**89**:398-404. DOI: 10.1016/j.tube.2009.07.004

[57] Hilda JN, Das S, Tripathy SP, Hanna LE. Role of Neutrophils in Tuberculosis: A Bird's Eye View. Vol. 26. London, England: SAGE Publications; 2020. pp. 240-247

[58] Yang CT, Cambier CJ, Davis JM, Hall CJ, Crosier PS, Ramakrishnan L. Neutrophils exert protection in the early tuberculous granuloma by oxidative killing of mycobacteria phagocytosed from infected macrophages. Cell Host & Microbe. 2012;**12**:301-312. DOI: 10.1016/j.chom.2012.07.009

[59] Niazi MKK, Dhulekar N, Schmidt D, Major S, Cooper R, Abeijon C, et al. Lung necrosis and neutrophils reflect common pathways of susceptibility to *Mycobacterium tuberculosis* in genetically diverse, immune-competent mice. Disease Models & Mechanisms. 2015;**8**:1141-1153. DOI: 10.1242/dmm.020867

[60] Dallenga T, Repnik U, Corleis B, Eich J, Reimer R, Griffiths GW, et al. *M. tuberculosis*-induced necrosis of infected neutrophils promotes bacterial growth following phagocytosis by macrophages. Cell Host & Microbe. 2017;**22**:519-530. DOI: 10.1016/j.chom.2017.09.003

[61] Lowe DM, Bandara AK, Packe GE, Barker RD, Wilkinson RJ, Griffiths CJ, et al. Neutrophilia independently predicts death in tuberculosis. The European Respiratory Journal. 2013;**42**:1752-1757. DOI: 10.1183/09031936.00140913

[62] Hult C, Mattila JT, Gideon HP, Linderman JJ, Kirschner DE. Neutrophil dynamics affect *Mycobacterium tuberculosis* granuloma outcomes and dissemination. Frontiers in Immunology. 2021;**12**:712457. DOI: 10.3389/fimmu.2021.712457

[63] Cong J, Wei H. Natural killer cells in the lungs. Frontiers in Immunology. 2019;**10**:1416. DOI: 10.3389/fimmu.2019.01416

[64] Choreno PJ, Martinez ZN, Jimenez ZL, Jimenez AL, Salinas LC, Zuniga J. Memory of natural killer cells: A new chance against *Mycobacterium tuberculosis*? Frontiers in Immunology. 2017;**8**:967. DOI: 10.3389/fimmu.2017.00967

[65] Abebe F. Immunological basis of early clearance of *Mycobacterium tuberculosis* infection: The role of natural killer cells. Clinical and Experimental Immunology. 2021;**204**:32-40. DOI: 10.1111/cei.13565

[66] Qin Y, Wang Q, Shi J. Immune checkpoint modulating T cells and NK cells response to *Mycobacterium tuberculosis* infection. Microbiological Research. 2023;**273**:127393. DOI: 10.1016/j.micres.2023.127393

[67] Garand M, Goodier M, Owolabi O, Donkor S, Kampmann B, Sutherland JS. Functional and phenotypic changes of natural killer cells in whole blood during *Mycobacterium tuberculosis*

infection and disease. Frontiers in Immunology. 2018;**9**:257. DOI: 10.3389/fimmu.2018.00257

[68] Esin S, Batoni G, Counoupas C, Stringaro A, Brancatisano FL, Colone M, et al. Direct binding of human NK cell natural cytotoxicity receptor NKp44 to the surfaces of mycobacteria and other bacteria. Infection and Immunity. 2008;**76**:1719-1727. DOI: 10.1128/iai.00870-07

[69] Gideon HP, Hughes TK, Tzouanas CN, Wadsworth MH, Tu AA, Gierahn TM, et al. Multimodal profiling of lung granulomas in macaques reveals cellular correlates of tuberculosis control. Immunity (Cambridge, Mass.). 2022;**55**:827-846. DOI: 10.1016/j.immuni.2022.04.004

[70] Feng CG, Kaviratne M, Rothfuchs AG, Cheever A, Hieny S, Young HA, et al. NK cell-derived IFN-gamma differentially regulates innate resistance and neutrophil response in T cell-deficient hosts infected with *Mycobacterium tuberculosis*. Journal of Immunology. 2006;**177**:7086-7093. DOI: 10.4049/jimmunol.177.10.7086

[71] Junqueira-Kipnis AP, Kipnis A, Jamieson A, Juarrero MG, Diefenbach A, Raulet DH, et al. NK cells respond to pulmonary infection with *Mycobacterium tuberculosis*, but play a minimal role in protection. Journal of Immunology. 2003;**171**:6039-6045. DOI: 10.4049/jimmunol.171.11.6039

[72] Allen M, Bailey C, Cahatol I, Dodge L, Yim J, Kassissa C, et al. Mechanisms of control of *Mycobacterium tuberculosis* by NK cells: Role of glutathione. Frontiers in Immunology. 2015;**6**:508. DOI: 10.3389/fimmu.2015.00508

[73] Gaffney E, Murphy D, Walsh A, Connolly S, Basdeo SA, Keane J, et al. Defining the role of neutrophils in the lung during infection: Implications for tuberculosis disease. Frontiers in Immunology. 2022;**13**:984293. DOI: 10.3389/fimmu.2022.984293

[74] Esin S, Batoni G. Natural killer cells: A coherent model for their functional role in *Mycobacterium tuberculosis* infection. Journal of Innate Immunity. 2015;**7**:11-24. DOI: 10.1159/000363321

[75] Murphy M, Suliman S, Briel L, Veldtsman H, Khomba N, Africa H, et al. Newborn bacille Calmette-Guerin vaccination induces robust infant interferon-gamma-expressing natural killer cell responses to mycobacteria. International Journal of Infectious Diseases. 2023;**130**(Suppl. 1):S52-S62. DOI: 10.1016/j.ijid.2023.02.018

[76] Suliman S, Geldenhuys H, Johnson JL, Hughes JE, Smit E, Murphy M, et al. Bacillus Calmette-Guerin (BCG) revaccination of adults with latent *Mycobacterium tuberculosis* infection induces long-lived BCG-reactive NK cell responses. Journal of Immunology. 2016;**197**:1100-1110. DOI: 10.4049/jimmunol.1501996

[77] Bowdish DM, Sakamoto K, Kim MJ, Kroos M, Mukhopadhyay S, Leifer CA, et al. MARCO, TLR2, and CD14 are required for macrophage cytokine responses to mycobacterial trehalose dimycolate and *Mycobacterium tuberculosis*. PLoS Pathogens. 2009;**5**:e1000474. DOI: 10.1371/journal.ppat.1000474

[78] Saiga H, Kitada S, Shimada Y, Kamiyama N, Okuyama M, Makino M, et al. Critical role of AIM2 in *Mycobacterium tuberculosis* infection. International Immunology. 2012;**24**:637-644. DOI: 10.1093/intimm/dxs062

[79] Moura-Alves P, Fae K, Houthuys E, Dorhoi A, Kreuchwig A, Furkert J,

et al. AhR sensing of bacterial pigments regulates antibacterial defence. Nature. 2014;**512**:387-392. DOI: 10.1038/nature13684

[80] Campos PC, Cunha DT, Souza-Costa LP, Shiloh MU, Franco LH. Bag it, tag it: Ubiquitin ligases and host resistance to *Mycobacterium tuberculosis*. Trends in Microbiology. 2022;**30**:973-985. DOI: 10.1016/j.tim.2022.03.010

[81] Kawai T, Akira S. The role of pattern-recognition receptors in innate immunity: Update on toll-like receptors. Nature Immunology. 2010;**11**:373-384. DOI: 10.1038/ni.1863

[82] Drennan MB, Nicolle D, Quesniaux VJ, Jacobs M, Allie N, Mpagi J, et al. Toll-like receptor 2-deficient mice succumb to *Mycobacterium tuberculosis* infection. The American Journal of Pathology. 2004;**164**:49-57. DOI: 10.1016/S0002-9440(10)63095-7

[83] Lai YF, Lin TM, Wang CH, Su PY, Wu JT, Lin MC, et al. Functional polymorphisms of the TLR7 and TLR8 genes contribute to *Mycobacterium tuberculosis* infection. Tuberculosis (Edinburgh, Scotland). 2016;**98**:125-131. DOI: 10.1016/j.tube.2016.03.008

[84] Carvalho NB, Oliveira FS, Duraes FV, de Almeida LA, Florido M, Prata LO, et al. Toll-like receptor 9 is required for full host resistance to *Mycobacterium avium* infection but plays no role in induction of Th1 responses. Infection and Immunity. 2011;**79**:1638-1646. DOI: 10.1128/IAI.01030-10

[85] Holscher C, Reiling N, Schaible UE, Holscher A, Bathmann C, Korbel D, et al. Containment of aerogenic *Mycobacterium tuberculosis* infection in mice does not require MyD88 adaptor function for TLR2, -4 and -9. European Journal of Immunology. 2008;**38**:680-694. DOI: 10.1002/eji.200736458

[86] Mayer-Barber KD, Barber DL, Shenderov K, White SD, Wilson MS, Cheever A, et al. Caspase-1 independent IL-1beta production is critical for host resistance to *mycobacterium tuberculosis* and does not require TLR signaling in vivo. Journal of Immunology. 2010;**184**:3326-3330. DOI: 10.4049/jimmunol. 0904189

[87] Pecora ND, Gehring AJ, Canaday DH, Boom WH, Harding CV. *Mycobacterium tuberculosis* LprA is a lipoprotein agonist of TLR2 that regulates innate immunity and APC function. Journal of Immunology. 2006;**177**:422-429. DOI: 10.4049/jimmunol.177.1.422

[88] Bai W, Liu H, Ji Q, Zhou Y, Liang L, Zheng R, et al. TLR3 regulates mycobacterial RNA-induced IL-10 production through the PI3K/AKT signaling pathway. Cellular Signalling. 2014;**26**:942-950. DOI: 10.1016/j.cellsig.2014.01.015

[89] Liu Y, Li JY, Chen ST, Huang HR, Cai H. The rLrp of *Mycobacterium tuberculosis* inhibits proinflammatory cytokine production and downregulates APC function in mouse macrophages via a TLR2-mediated PI3K/Akt pathway activation-dependent mechanism. Cellular & Molecular Immunology. 2016;**13**:729-746. DOI: 10.1038/cmi.2015.58

[90] Su H, Zhang Z, Liu Z, Peng B, Kong C, Wang H, et al. *Mycobacterium tuberculosis* PPE60 antigen drives Th1/Th17 responses via toll-like receptor 2-dependent maturation of dendritic cells. The Journal of Biological Chemistry. 2018;**293**:10287-10302. DOI: 10.1074/jbc.RA118.001696

[91] Wang J, Li BX, Ge PP, Li J, Wang Q, Gao GF, et al. *Mycobacterium tuberculosis*

suppresses innate immunity by coopting the host ubiquitin system. Nature Immunology. 2015;**16**:237-245. DOI: 10.1038/ni.3096

[92] Li J, Chai QY, Zhang Y, Li BX, Wang J, Qiu XB, et al. *Mycobacterium tuberculosis* Mce3E suppresses host innate immune responses by targeting ERK1/2 signaling. Journal of Immunology. 2015;**194**:3756-3767. DOI: 10.4049/jimmunol.1402679

[93] Khan N, Pahari S, Vidyarthi A, Aqdas M, Agrewala JN. Stimulation through CD40 and TLR-4 is an effective host directed therapy against *Mycobacterium tuberculosis*. Frontiers in Immunology. 2016;7:386. DOI: 10.3389/fimmu.2016.00386

[94] Simeone R, Bobard A, Lippmann J, Bitter W, Majlessi L, Brosch R, et al. Phagosomal rupture by *Mycobacterium tuberculosis* results in toxicity and host cell death. PLoS Pathogens. 2012;**8**:e1002507. DOI: 10.1371/journal.ppat.1002507

[95] Juarez E, Carranza C, Hernandez-Sanchez F, Leon-Contreras JC, Hernandez-Pando R, Escobedo D, et al. NOD2 enhances the innate response of alveolar macrophages to *Mycobacterium tuberculosis* in humans. European Journal of Immunology. 2012;**42**:880-889. DOI: 10.1002/eji.201142105

[96] Austin CM, Ma X, Graviss EA. Common nonsynonymous polymorphisms in the NOD2 gene are associated with resistance or susceptibility to tuberculosis disease in African Americans. The Journal of Infectious Diseases. 2008;**197**:1713-1716. DOI: 10.1086/588384

[97] Yang Y, Xu P, He P, Shi F, Tang Y, Guan C, et al. Mycobacterial PPE13 activates inflammasome by interacting with the NATCH and LRR domains of NLRP3. The FASEB Journal. 2020;**34**:12820-12833. DOI: 10.1096/fj.202000200RR

[98] Qu Z, Zhou J, Zhou Y, Xie Y, Jiang Y, Wu J, et al. Mycobacterial EST12 activates a RACK1-NLRP3-gasdermin D pyroptosis-IL-1β immune pathway. Science Advances. 2020;**6**:eaba4733. DOI: 10.1126/sciadv.aba4733

[99] Xu F, Qi H, Li J, Sun L, Gong J, Chen Y, et al. *Mycobacterium tuberculosis* infection upregulates MFN2 expression to promote NLRP3 inflammasome formation. The Journal of Biological Chemistry. 2020;**295**:17684-17697. DOI: 10.1074/jbc.RA120.014077

[100] Zhang J, Cui Y, Zang X, Feng T, Chen F, Wang H, et al. PE12 interaction with TLR4 promotes intracellular survival of *Mycobacterium tuberculosis* by suppressing inflammatory response. International Journal of Biological Macromolecules. 2023;**253**:127547. DOI: 10.1016/j.ijbiomac. 2023.127547

[101] Rastogi S, Ellinwood S, Augenstreich J, Mayer-Barber KD, Briken V, Behr MA. *Mycobacterium tuberculosis* inhibits the NLRP3 inflammasome activation via its phosphokinase PknF. PLoS Pathogens. 2021;**17**:e1009712. DOI: 10.1371/journal.ppat.1009712

[102] Goyal S, Klassert TE, Slevogt H. C-type lectin receptors in tuberculosis: What we know. Medical Microbiology and Immunology. 2016;**205**:513-535. DOI: 10.1007/s00430-016-0470-1

[103] Kang PB, Azad AK, Torrelles JB, Kaufman TM, Beharka A, Tibesar E, et al. The human macrophage mannose receptor directs *Mycobacterium tuberculosis* lipoarabinomannan-mediated phagosome biogenesis. The

Journal of Experimental Medicine. 2005;**202**:987-999. DOI: 10.1084/jem.20051239

[104] Lugo-Villarino G, Troegeler A, Balboa L, Lastrucci C, Duval C, Mercier I, et al. The C-type lectin receptor DC-SIGN has an anti-inflammatory role in human M(IL-4) macrophages in response to *Mycobacterium tuberculosis*. Frontiers in Immunology. 2018;**9**:1123. DOI: 10.3389/fimmu.2018.01123

[105] Yadav M, Schorey JS. The beta-glucan receptor dectin-1 functions together with TLR2 to mediate macrophage activation by mycobacteria. Blood. 2006;**108**:3168-3175. DOI: 10.1182/blood-2006-05-024406

[106] Yonekawa A, Saijo S, Hoshino Y, Miyake Y, Ishikawa E, Suzukawa M, et al. Dectin-2 is a direct receptor for mannose-capped lipoarabinomannan of mycobacteria. Immunity. 2014;**41**:402-413. DOI: 10.1016/j.immuni.2014.08.005

[107] Miyake Y, Masatsugu OH, Yamasaki S. C-type lectin receptor MCL facilitates mincle expression and signaling through complex formation. Journal of Immunology. 2015;**194**:5366-5374. DOI: 10.4049/jimmunol.1402429

[108] Troegeler A, Lugo-Villarino G, Hansen S, Rasolofo V, Henriksen ML, Mori K, et al. Collectin CL-LK is a novel soluble pattern recognition receptor for *Mycobacterium tuberculosis*. PLoS ONE. 2015;**10**:e132692. DOI: 10.1371/journal.pone.0132692

[109] Troegeler A, Mercier I, Cougoule C, Pietretti D, Colom A, Duval C, et al. C-type lectin receptor DCIR modulates immunity to tuberculosis by sustaining type I interferon signaling in dendritic cells. Proceedings of the National Academy of Sciences of the United States of America. 2017;**114**:E540-E549. DOI: 10.1073/pnas.1613254114

[110] Korb VC, Chuturgoon AA, Moodley D. *Mycobacterium tuberculosis*: Manipulator of protective immunity. International Journal of Molecular Sciences. 2016;**17**:131. DOI: 10.3390/ijms17030131

[111] Hmama Z, Pena-Diaz S, Joseph S, Av-Gay Y. Immunoevasion and immunosuppression of the macrophage by *Mycobacterium tuberculosis*. Immunological Reviews. 2015;**264**:220-232. DOI: 10.1111/imr.12268

[112] Vergne I, Fratti RA, Hill PJ, Chua J, Belisle J, Deretic V. *Mycobacterium tuberculosis* phagosome maturation arrest: Mycobacterial phosphatidylinositol analog phosphatidylinositol mannoside stimulates early endosomal fusion. Molecular Biology of the Cell. 2004;**15**:751-760. DOI: 10.1091/mbc.e03-05-0307

[113] Kyei GB, Vergne I, Chua J, Roberts E, Harris J, Junutula JR, et al. Rab14 is critical for maintenance of *Mycobacterium tuberculosis* phagosome maturation arrest. The EMBO Journal. 2006;**25**:5250-5259. DOI: 10.1038/sj.emboj.7601407

[114] Ehlers S. DC-SIGN and mannosylated surface structures of *Mycobacterium tuberculosis*: A deceptive liaison. European Journal of Cell Biology. 2010;**89**:95-101. DOI: 10.1016/j.ejcb.2009.10.004

[115] Walburger A, Koul A, Ferrari G, Nguyen L, Prescianotto-Baschong C, Huygen K, et al. Protein kinase G from pathogenic mycobacteria promotes survival within macrophages. Science. 2004;**304**:1800-1804. DOI: 10.1126/science.1099384

[116] Wong D, Bach H, Sun J, Hmama Z, Av-Gay Y. *Mycobacterium tuberculosis* protein tyrosine phosphatase (PtpA) excludes host vacuolar-H+-ATPase to inhibit phagosome acidification. Proceedings of the National Academy of Sciences of the United States of America. 2011;**108**:19371-19376. DOI: 10.1073/pnas.1109201108

[117] Abramovitch RB, Rohde KH, Hsu FF, Russell DG. aprABC: A *Mycobacterium tuberculosis* complex-specific locus that modulates pH-driven adaptation to the macrophage phagosome. Molecular Microbiology. 2011;**80**:678-694. DOI: 10.1111/j.1365-2958.2011.07601.x

[118] Wee YS, Roundy KM, Weis JJ, Weis JH. Interferon-inducible transmembrane proteins of the innate immune response act as membrane organizers by influencing clathrin and v-ATPase localization and function. Innate Immunity (London, England). 2012;**18**:834-845. DOI: 10.1177/1753425912443392

[119] Liu M, Li W, Xiang X, Xie J. *Mycobacterium tuberculosis* effectors interfering host apoptosis signaling. Apoptosis. 2015;**20**:883-891. DOI: 10.1007/s10495-015-1115-3

[120] Winau F, Weber S, Sad S, de Diego J, Hoops SL, Breiden B, et al. Apoptotic vesicles crossprime CD8 T cells and protect against tuberculosis. Immunity. 2006;**24**:105-117. DOI: 10.1016/j.immuni.2005.12.001

[121] Poirier V, Bach H, Av-Gay Y. *Mycobacterium tuberculosis* promotes anti-apoptotic activity of the macrophage by PtpA protein-dependent dephosphorylation of host GSK3alpha. The Journal of Biological Chemistry. 2014;**289**:29376-29385. DOI: 10.1074/jbc.M114.582502

[122] Velmurugan K, Chen B, Miller JL, Azogue S, Gurses S, Hsu T, et al. *Mycobacterium tuberculosis* nuoG is a virulence gene that inhibits apoptosis of infected host cells. PLoS Pathogens. 2007;**3**:e110. DOI: 10.1371/journal.ppat.0030110

[123] Molle V, Girard-Blanc C, Kremer L, Doublet P, Cozzone AJ, Prost JF. Protein PknE, a novel transmembrane eukaryotic-like serine/threonine kinase from *Mycobacterium tuberculosis*. Biochemical and Biophysical Research Communications. 2003;**308**:820-825. DOI: 10.1016/s0006-291x(03)01476-1

[124] Hinchey J, Lee S, Jeon BY, Basaraba RJ, Venkataswamy MM, Chen B, et al. Enhanced priming of adaptive immunity by a proapoptotic mutant of *Mycobacterium tuberculosis*. The Journal of Clinical Investigation. 2007;**117**:2279-2288. DOI: 10.1172/JCI31947

[125] Jain R, Dey B, Khera A, Srivastav P, Gupta UD, Katoch VM, et al. Over-expression of superoxide dismutase obliterates the protective effect of BCG against tuberculosis by modulating innate and adaptive immune responses. Vaccine. 2011;**29**:8118-8125. DOI: 10.1016/j.vaccine.2011.08.029

[126] Dutta NK, Mehra S, Martinez AN, Alvarez X, Renner NA, Morici LA, et al. The stress-response factor SigH modulates the interaction between *Mycobacterium tuberculosis* and host phagocytes. PLoS ONE. 2012;**7**:e28958. DOI: 10.1371/journal.pone.0028958

[127] Wang Q, Liu S, Tang Y, Liu Q, Yao Y. MPT64 protein from *Mycobacterium tuberculosis* inhibits apoptosis of macrophages through NF-kB-miRNA21-Bcl-2 pathway. PLoS ONE. 2014;**9**:e100949. DOI: 10.1371/journal.pone.0100949

[128] Danelishvili L, Babrak L, Rose SJ, Everman J, Bermudez LE, Kaufmann SHE. *Mycobacterium tuberculosis* alters the metalloprotease activity of the COP9 signalosome. MBio. 2014;**5**:e01278-14. DOI: 10.1128/mBio.01278-14

[129] Joseph S, Yuen A, Singh V, Hmama Z. *Mycobacterium tuberculosis* Cpn60.2 (GroEL2) blocks macrophage apoptosis via interaction with mitochondrial mortalin. Biology Open. 2017;**6**:481-488. DOI: 10.1242/bio.023119

[130] Jurcic SK, Lee S. Inhibition of apoptosis by Rv2456c through nuclear factor-kappaB extends the survival of *Mycobacterium tuberculosis*. International Journal of Mycobacteriology. 2016;**5**:426-436. DOI: 10.1016/j.ijmyco.2016.06.018

[131] Xu G, Jia H, Li Y, Liu X, Li M, Wang Y. Hemolytic phospholipase Rv0183 of *Mycobacterium tuberculosis* induces inflammatory response and apoptosis in alveolar macrophage RAW264.7 cells. Canadian Journal of Microbiology. 2010;**56**:916-924. DOI: 10.1139/w10-079

[132] Sanchez A, Espinosa P, Esparza MA, Colon M, Bernal G, Mancilla R. *Mycobacterium tuberculosis* 38-kDa lipoprotein is apoptogenic for human monocyte-derived macrophages. Scandinavian Journal of Immunology. 2009;**69**:20-28. DOI: 10.1111/j.1365-3083.2008.02193.x

[133] Dasgupta A, Sureka K, Mitra D, Saha B, Sanyal S, Das AK, et al. An oligopeptide transporter of *Mycobacterium tuberculosis* regulates cytokine release and apoptosis of infected macrophages. PLoS ONE. 2010;**5**:e12225. DOI: 10.1371/journal.pone.0012225

[134] Samten B, Wang X, Barnes PF. *Mycobacterium tuberculosis* ESX-1 system-secreted protein ESAT-6 but not CFP10 inhibits human T-cell immune responses. Tuberculosis (Edinburgh, Scotland). 2009;**89**(Suppl. 1):S74-S76. DOI: 10.1016/S1472-9792(09)70017-4

[135] Balaji KN, Goyal G, Narayana Y, Srinivas M, Chaturvedi R, Mohammad S. Apoptosis triggered by Rv1818c, a PE family gene from *Mycobacterium tuberculosis* is regulated by mitochondrial intermediates in T cells. Microbes and Infection. 2007;**9**:271-281. DOI: 10.1016/j.micinf.2006.11.013

[136] Lopez M, Sly LM, Luu Y, Young D, Cooper H, Reiner NE. The 19-kDa *Mycobacterium tuberculosis* protein induces macrophage apoptosis through toll-like receptor-2. Journal of Immunology. 2003;**170**:2409-2416. DOI: 10.4049/jimmunol.170.5.2409

[137] Tiwari B, Ramakrishnan UM, Raghunand TR. The *Mycobacterium tuberculosis* protein pair PE9 (Rv1088)-PE10 (Rv1089) forms heterodimers and induces macrophage apoptosis through toll-like receptor 4. Cellular Microbiology. 2015;**17**:1653-1669. DOI: 10.1111/cmi.12462

[138] Saini NK, Sinha R, Singh P, Sharma M, Pathak R, Rathor N, et al. Mce4A protein of *Mycobacterium tuberculosis* induces pro inflammatory cytokine response leading to macrophage apoptosis in a TNF-α dependent manner. Microbial Pathogenesis. 2016;**100**:43-50. DOI: 10.1016/j.micpath.2016.08.038

[139] Ciaramella A, Martino A, Cicconi R, Colizzi V, Fraziano M. Mycobacterial 19-kDa lipoprotein mediates *Mycobacterium tuberculosis*-induced apoptosis in monocytes/macrophages at early stages of infection. Cell Death and Differentiation. 2000;**7**:1270-1272. DOI: 10.1038/sj.cdd.4400761

[140] Ahmad J, Farhana A, Pancsa R, Arora SK, Srinivasan A, Tyagi AK, et al. Contrasting function of structured N-terminal and unstructured C-terminal segments of *Mycobacterium tuberculosis* PPE37 protein. MBio. 2018;**9**:e01712-17. DOI: 10.1128/mBio.01712-17

[141] Deng W, Long Q, Zeng J, Li P, Yang W, Chen X, et al. *Mycobacterium tuberculosis* PE_PGRS41 enhances the intracellular survival of *M. smegmatis* within macrophages via blocking innate immunity and inhibition of host defense. Scientific Reports. 2017;**7**:46716. DOI: 10.1038/srep46716

[142] Li H, Li Q, Yu Z, Zhou M, Xie J. *Mycobacterium tuberculosis* PE13 (Rv1195) manipulates the host cell fate via p38-ERK-NF-kappaB axis and apoptosis. Apoptosis. 2016;**21**:795-808. DOI: 10.1007/s10495-016-1249-y

[143] Yang W, Deng W, Zeng J, Ren S, Ali MK, Gu Y, et al. *Mycobacterium tuberculosis* PE_PGRS18 enhances the intracellular survival of *M. smegmatis* via altering host macrophage cytokine profiling and attenuating the cell apoptosis. Apoptosis. 2017;**22**:502-509. DOI: 10.1007/s10495-016-1336-0

[144] Palucci I, Camassa S, Cascioferro A, Sali M, Anoosheh S, Zumbo A, et al. PE_PGRS33 contributes to *Mycobacterium tuberculosis* entry in macrophages through interaction with TLR2. PLoS ONE. 2016;**11**:e150800. DOI: 10.1371/journal.pone.0150800

[145] Mizushima N, Levine B. Autophagy in human diseases. The New England Journal of Medicine. 2020;**383**:1564-1576. DOI: 10.1056/NEJMra2022774

[146] Kim YS, Silwal P, Kim SY, Yoshimori T, Jo EK. Autophagy-activating strategies to promote innate defense against mycobacteria. Experimental & Molecular Medicine. 2019;**51**:1-10. DOI: 10.1038/s12276-019-0290-7

[147] Paik S, Kim JK, Chung C, Jo EK. Autophagy: A new strategy for host-directed therapy of tuberculosis. Virulence. 2019;**10**:448-459. DOI: 10.1080/21505594.2018.1536598

[148] Watson RO, Manzanillo PS, Cox JS, Extracellular M. Tuberculosis DNA targets bacteria for autophagy by activating the host DNA-sensing pathway. Cell. 2012;**150**:803-815. DOI: 10.1016/j.cell.2012.06.040

[149] Dutta RK, Kathania M, Raje M, Majumdar S. IL-6 inhibits IFN-gamma induced autophagy in *Mycobacterium tuberculosis* H37Rv infected macrophages. The International Journal of Biochemistry & Cell Biology. 2012;**44**:942-954. DOI: 10.1016/j.biocel.2012.02.021

[150] Seto S, Tsujimura K, Horii T, Koide Y. Autophagy adaptor protein p62/SQSTM1 and autophagy-related gene Atg5 mediate autophagosome formation in response to *Mycobacterium tuberculosis* infection in dendritic cells. PLoS ONE. 2013;**8**:e86017. DOI: 10.1371/journal.pone.0086017

[151] Gutierrez MG, Master SS, Singh SB, Taylor GA, Colombo MI, Deretic V. Autophagy is a defense mechanism inhibiting BCG and *Mycobacterium tuberculosis* survival in infected macrophages. Cell. 2004;**119**:753-766. DOI: 10.1016/j.cell.2004.11.038

[152] Wang J, Yang K, Zhou L, Minhaowu WY, Zhu M, Lai X, et al. MicroRNA-155 promotes autophagy to eliminate intracellular mycobacteria by targeting Rheb. PLoS Pathogens. 2013;**9**:e1003697. DOI: 10.1371/journal.ppat.1003697

[153] Kimmey JM, Huynh JP, Weiss LA, Park S, Kambal A, Debnath J, et al. Unique role for ATG5 in neutrophil-mediated immunopathology during *M. tuberculosis* infection. Nature. 2015;**528**:565-569. DOI: 10.1038/nature16451

[154] Castillo EF, Dekonenko A, Arko-Mensah J, Mandell MA, Dupont N, Jiang S, et al. Autophagy protects against active tuberculosis by suppressing bacterial burden and inflammation. Proceedings of the National Academy of Sciences of the United States of America. 2012;**109**:E3168-E3176. DOI: 10.1073/pnas.1210500109

[155] Xu Y, Fattah EA, Liu XD, Jagannath C, Eissa NT. Harnessing of TLR-mediated autophagy to combat mycobacteria in macrophages. Tuberculosis (Edinburgh, Scotland). 2013;**93**(Suppl.):S33-S37. DOI: 10.1016/S1472-9792(13)70008-8

[156] Singh SB, Davis AS, Taylor GA, Deretic V. Human IRGM induces autophagy to eliminate intracellular mycobacteria. Science. 2006;**313**:1438-1441. DOI: 10.1126/science.1129577

[157] Yuan L, Ke Z, Ma J, Guo Y, Li Y. IRGM gene polymorphisms and haplotypes associate with susceptibility of pulmonary tuberculosis in Chinese Hubei Han population. Tuberculosis (Edinburgh, Scotland). 2016;**96**:58-64. DOI: 10.1016/j.tube.2015.10.014

[158] Lu Y, Li Q, Peng J, Zhu Y, Wang F, Wang C, et al. Association of autophagy-related IRGM polymorphisms with latent versus active tuberculosis infection in a Chinese population. Tuberculosis (Edinburgh, Scotland). 2016;**97**:47-51. DOI: 10.1016/j.tube.2016.01.001

[159] Dey B, Dey RJ, Cheung LS, Pokkali S, Guo H, Lee JH, et al. A bacterial cyclic dinucleotide activates the cytosolic surveillance pathway and mediates innate resistance to tuberculosis. Nature Medicine. 2015;**21**:401-406. DOI: 10.1038/nm.3813

[160] Via LE, Deretic D, Ulmer RJ, Hibler NS, Huber LA, Deretic V. Arrest of mycobacterial phagosome maturation is caused by a block in vesicle fusion between stages controlled by rab5 and rab7. The Journal of Biological Chemistry. 1997;**272**:13326-13331. DOI: 10.1074/jbc.272.20.13326

[161] Roberts EA, Chua J, Kyei GB, Deretic V. Higher order Rab programming in phagolysosome biogenesis. The Journal of Cell Biology. 2006;**174**:923-929. DOI: 10.1083/jcb.200603026

[162] Cardoso CM, Jordao L, Vieira OV. Rab10 regulates phagosome maturation and its overexpression rescues Mycobacterium-containing phagosomes maturation. Traffic. 2010;**11**:221-235. DOI: 10.1111/j.1600-0854.2009.01013.x

[163] Zhang L, Zhang H, Zhao Y, Mao F, Wu J, Bai B, et al. Effects of *Mycobacterium tuberculosis* ESAT-6/CFP-10 fusion protein on the autophagy function of mouse macrophages. DNA and Cell Biology. 2012;**31**:171-179. DOI: 10.1089/dna.2011.1290

[164] Kim KH, An DR, Song J, Yoon JY, Kim HS, Yoon HJ, et al. *Mycobacterium tuberculosis* Eis protein initiates suppression of host immune responses by acetylation of DUSP16/MKP-7. Proceedings of the National Academy of Sciences of the United States of America. 2012;**109**:7729-7734. DOI: 10.1073/pnas.1120251109

[165] Puri RV, Reddy PV, Tyagi AK. Secreted acid phosphatase (SapM) of *Mycobacterium tuberculosis* is

indispensable for arresting phagosomal maturation and growth of the pathogen in guinea pig tissues. PLoS ONE. 2013;**8**:e70514. DOI: 10.1371/journal.pone.0070514

[166] Vazquez CL, Bianco MV, Blanco FC, Forrellad MA, Gutierrez MG, Bigi F. *Mycobacterium bovis* requires P27 (LprG) to arrest phagosome maturation and replicate within bovine macrophages. Infection and Immunity. 2017;**85**:e00720-16. DOI: 10.1128/IAI.00720-16

[167] Quigley J, Hughitt VK, Velikovsky CA, Mariuzza RA, El-Sayed NM, Briken V. The cell wall lipid PDIM contributes to phagosomal escape and host cell exit of *Mycobacterium tuberculosis*. MBio. 2017;**8**:e00148-17. DOI: 10.1128/mBio.00148-17

[168] Man SM, Karki R, Kanneganti TD. Molecular mechanisms and functions of pyroptosis, inflammatory caspases and inflammasomes in infectious diseases. Immunological Reviews. 2017;**277**:61-75. DOI: 10.1111/imr.12534

[169] Huang Y, Xu W, Zhou R. NLRP3 inflammasome activation and cell death. Cellular & Molecular Immunology. 2021;**18**:2114-2127. DOI: 10.1038/s41423-021-00740-6

[170] Beckwith KS, Beckwith MS, Ullmann S, Saetra RS, Kim H, Marstad A, et al. Plasma membrane damage causes NLRP3 activation and pyroptosis during *Mycobacterium tuberculosis* infection. Nature Communications. 2020;**11**:2270. DOI: 10.1038/s41467-020-16143-6

[171] Basu S, Fowler BJ, Kerur N, Arnvig KB, Rao NA. NLRP3 inflammasome activation by mycobacterial ESAT-6 and dsRNA in intraocular tuberculosis. Microbial Pathogenesis. 2018;**114**:219-224. DOI: 10.1016/j.micpath.2017.11.044

[172] Ma J, Zhao S, Gao X, Wang R, Liu J, Zhou X, et al. The roles of inflammasomes in host defense against *Mycobacterium tuberculosis*. Pathogens. 2021;**10**:120. DOI: 10.3390/pathogens10020120

[173] Yang E, Yang R, Guo M, Huang D, Wang W, Zhang Z, et al. Multidrug-resistant tuberculosis (MDR-TB) strain infection in macaques results in high bacilli burdens in airways, driving broad innate/adaptive immune responses. Emerging Microbes & Infections. 2018;**7**:207. DOI: 10.1038/s41426-018-0213-z

[174] Howard NC, Khader SA. Immunometabolism during *Mycobacterium tuberculosis* infection. Trends in Microbiology. 2020;**28**:832-850. DOI: 10.1016/j.tim.2020.04.010

[175] Howard NC, Marin ND, Ahmed M, Rosa BA, Martin J, Bambouskova M, et al. *Mycobacterium tuberculosis* carrying a rifampicin drug resistance mutation reprograms macrophage metabolism through cell wall lipid changes. Nature Microbiology. 2018;**3**:1099-1108. DOI: 10.1038/s41564-018-0245-0

[176] Cho HJ, Lim YJ, Kim J, Koh WJ, Song CH, Kang MW. Different macrophage polarization between drug-susceptible and multidrug-resistant pulmonary tuberculosis. BMC Infectious Diseases. 2020;**20**:81. DOI: 10.1186/s12879-020-4802-9

[177] Basingnaa A, Antwi-Baffour S, Nkansah DO, Afutu E, Owusu E. Plasma levels of cytokines (IL-10, IFN-gamma and TNF-alpha) in multidrug resistant tuberculosis and drug responsive tuberculosis patients in Ghana. Diseases. 2018;**7**:2. DOI: 10.3390/diseases7010002

[178] Romero MM, Basile JI, Lopez B, Ritacco V, Barrera L, Sasiain MC, et al. Outbreaks of *Mycobacterium tuberculosis* MDR strains differentially induce neutrophil respiratory burst involving lipid rafts, p38 MAPK and Syk. BMC Infectious Diseases. 2014;**14**:262. DOI: 10.1186/1471-2334-14-262

[179] Stutz MD, Allison CC, Ojaimi S, Preston SP, Doerflinger M, Arandjelovic P, et al. Macrophage and neutrophil death programs differentially confer resistance to tuberculosis. Immunity. 2021;**54**:1758-1771. DOI: 10.1016/j.immuni.2021.06.009

Chapter 3

The Expanding Antibiotic Resistance: The Requirement of New Therapeutic Strategy for the Development of New Anti-Infective

Saeid Besharati

Abstract

The spread of infectious diseases has increased, and without a doubt, the incorrect use and excessive use of antibiotics for human consumption, animal husbandry, and agriculture have been effective in the emergence of new infections and increased resistance to antibiotic treatment. Mechanisms of antibiotic resistance, such as biofilms, efflux pumps, and mutations in microorganisms, are some of the methods used by microorganisms to escape the host's immune system and develop antibiotic resistance in them. Our strategy for treatment should also be tailored to the adaptations made by microorganisms. We must look for new approaches to deal with pathogenic agents, new methods for treatment, as well as dealing with antibiotic resistance in them. Antimicrobial peptides, nanoparticles, and bacteriophage therapy in dealing with antibiotic resistance. In this chapter, we highlight the mechanisms of antibiotic resistance in bacteria and new approaches to deal with pathogens, and new methods for treatment.

Keywords: antimicrobial peptides, nanoparticles, bacteriophage therapy, immune cell, multidrug resistance, biofilm, efflux pump, treatment strategies

1. Introduction

Increasing consumption and misuse of antibiotics in human and veterinary cases has caused treatment failure and the spread of antibiotic resistance. This spread of resistance has been such that it is estimated that by 2050, about 10 million human deaths per year may be attributable to antimicrobial resistance. In recent years, the severe spread of infectious diseases and the spread of newly emerging diseases such as COVID-19 have increased these concerns [1–3]. Microorganisms from various mechanisms such as acquired genetic aspects and inherent and also, biochemical aspects such as biofilm formation, efflux pump, and change in membrane permeability accelerate the process of resistance to antibiotics and cause treatment failure due to MDR[1] in human patients and veterinary [4–7]. All these cases have caused widespread global concerns in dealing with microorganisms and have raised effective approaches to deal with them with the help of alternative tools. New strategies for dealing with microorganisms have been proposed as a suitable alternative to antibiotics, such as antimicrobial peptides, bacteriophages, and nanoparticles. Studies have reported positive results of alternative treatments to combat resistant microorganisms. In this chapter, we refer to the general review of the mechanisms and factors contributing to the emergence of resistance in microorganisms and alternative treatment approaches for antibiotics. We will discuss the advantages and limitations of the agents, considering alternative therapy applications, efficacy, development of resistance, and interactions with the immune system.

2. Mechanisms of resistance

Microorganisms use different mechanisms to resist antibiotics and evade host cell immunity, which can have biochemical or innate aspects (**Figure 1**). Undoubtedly, high selective toxicity in order to reduce complications for the host is one of the important characteristics of an ideal antimicrobial. Antibacterial classification is done based on the mechanism of action and target in the bacterial cell [8, 9]. Resistance mechanisms in microorganisms are very diverse and can be from different pathways such as biofilm formation, antibiotic efflux pumps and release systems, antibiotic enzyme inactivation, change in outer membrane permeability, change in target sites and purines, preventing drug access to specific targets (e.g., through reduced uptake

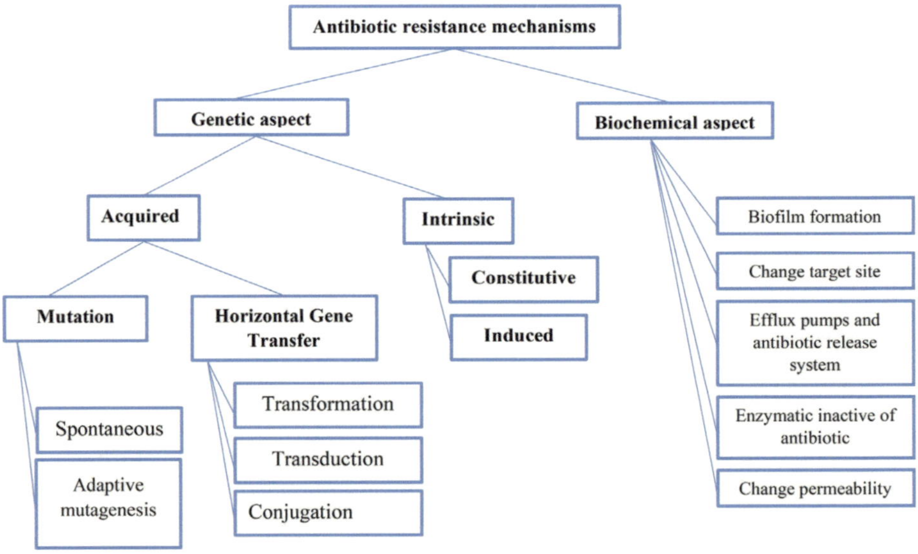

Figure 1.
Mechanisms of antibiotic resistance in microorganisms.

[1] Multi Drug Resistant.

by the cell through reduced permeability of the outer membrane (mutability) can be caused by spontaneous mutations, including genome and RNA changes). For example, rRNA mutations are associated with resistance to several antibiotics and horizontal gene transfer (Transformation, Transduction, and Conjugation) [10]. Resistance to antibiotics is not only acquired after exposure to it, and microorganisms can also have inherent resistance. Reducing the permeability of the outer membrane, biofilm formation to avoid exposure to antimicrobial agents, and efflux pumps are some of these things [11–13]. Acquired resistance is due to the acquisition of mobile resistance genes and chromosomal point mutations in resistant species. MGEs,[2] such as plasmids, bacteriophages, and integrons play an effective role in the emergence of MDR strains [14, 15].

2.1 Biofilm formation

Antonie van Leeuwenhoek first observed the formation of biofilm plaques on teeth more than 300 years ago. Costerton proposed the concept of biofilm in 1978, in the definition of biofilm, it can be said that the accumulation of cells on living or non-living surfaces with the formation of a matrix of biofilm polymer materials, which causes cells to be close to each other with high density until time suitable to transfer and expand [16, 17]. It is predicted that up to 80% of infections are related to biofilm formation or due to biofilm formation. Hospital infections with agents such as *Pseudomonas*, *Acinetobacter,* and other pathogens have become one of the most important health problems, which along with high resistance to antibiotics, can make the treatment process much more complicated [18–20].

2.1.1 Applications of biofilm

Biofilm acts like a double-edged sword, on the one hand, it can have useful applications such as the production of biofuels, living catalysts, bioremediation, purification of drinking water, and decomposition of waste in sewage, on the other hand, it can cause infection, antibiotic resistance, contamination of medical devices [21–24]. The EPS[3] matrix plays an important role in the development of biofilms and their resistance to various types of antibiotics [25]. Therefore, preventing the accumulation of EPS can be considered as an anti-biofilm agent, but in addition, other methods such as bacteriophage therapy, antimicrobial photodynamic for controlling bacterial biofilms and therapy (APDT) and cold atmospheric plasma (CAP), anti-biofilm peptides, photothermal therapy, nonthermal (cold) plasma, high-speed water micro spray to cause a physical disturbance, nanocoatings, etc. are considered as methods to prevent and inhibit biofilm (**Figure 2**) [26–29]. Therefore, our strategy is very important in interacting or dealing with biofilm. Despite the idea that biofilm formation can always be a problem, biofilm also has useful uses. Some applications of biofilm (microbial communities) include the purification of drinking water, the decomposition of waste into industrial, agricultural, and domestic wastewater, the disposal of dry waste, and they act as catalysts in biotechnological processes such as the production of biofuels (**Figure 3**) [21]. They can also be effective in producing quality agricultural products and reducing pest damage by inhibiting pests and plant

[2] Mobile Genetic Elements.

[3] Extracellular Polymeric Substances.

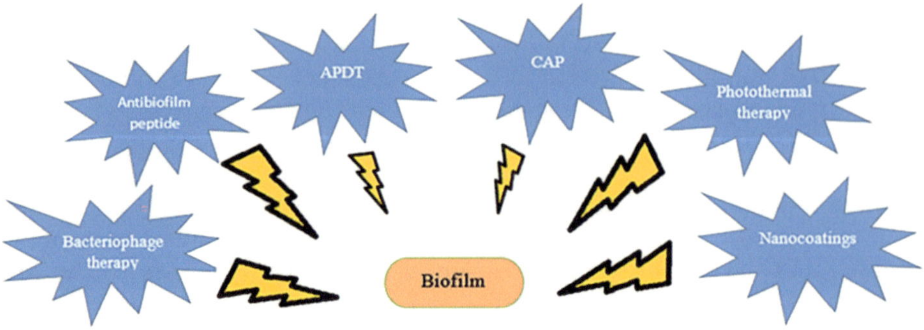

Figure 2.
Several pathways to combat with biofilm.

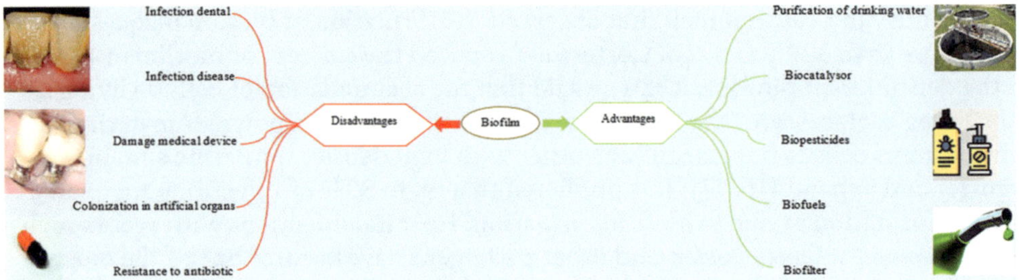

Figure 3.
Some of illustration of advantages and disadvantages of biofilm.

diseases [30]. Biofilm formation is not limited to living surfaces and can be found in a wide range of non-biological, plastic surfaces as well as medical devices and devices [31]. The use of contaminated medical devices can cause the formation of biofilm in the body, although accurate information on its amount and percentage is not available, it has been shown to cause infection in cases such as ventricular assist devices, joint prostheses, breast implants, pacemakers, and defibrillators, mechanical heart valves, ventricular shunts [32, 33]. Biofilm-related infections can occur in medical devices and equipment can cause a lot of costs and damages and may add more than $ 1 billion to the cost of hospitalized patients in the United States [32, 34]. Bacteria such as *P. aeruginosa,*[4] *E. coli,*[5] *Staphylococcus aureus*, can attach to ocular lenses and their storage boxes and biofilms formation [35–37].

2.1.2 Strategy to deal with biofilm

Anti-biofilm strategies are becoming more and more developed. In recent years, innovative and new methods have been developed to manage biofilm-related infections in the mouth, including antimicrobial photodynamics for controlling bacterial biofilms and therapy (APDT) and cold atmospheric plasma (CAP), which are effective in removing resistant biofilms (**Figure 4**) [17]. Anti-biofilm peptides that specifically target cariogenic agents [38], photothermal therapy, bacteriophages

[4] *Pseudomonas aeruginosa.*

[5] *Escherichia coli.*

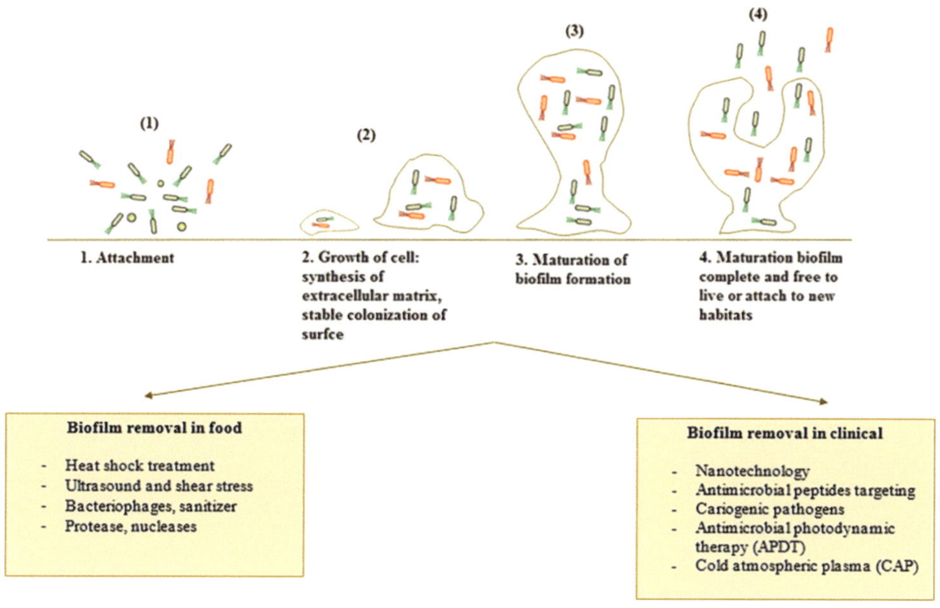

Figure 4.
Several steps of biofilm formation and method of removal biofilm in food and clinical sample.

therapy [39], nonthermal (cold) plasma [40, 41], high-speed water micro spray to cause a physical disturbance, nanocoatings, nanotechnology by activating stimuli and increasing selectivity, and controlled drug delivery at the biofilm site [42, 43]. The use of bacteria is effective in biologically controlling plant diseases and quantitatively and qualitatively improving the growth of agricultural products, and biofilms produced by beneficial bacteria such as *Bacillus subtilis* and *Pseudomonas fluorescent* can be effective in controlling plant diseases [44–46]. The biofilm formation in the environment, medical devices, drug resistance, and disease causes irreparable loss of life and property, which can be largely controlled by creating the right strategy.

2.1.3 Biofilms and evasion of immune responses

Biofilm infections are not exclusively surface phenomena, because they can penetrate deep into tissue and chronic wounds, such as *Mycobacterium ulcerans*. The adhesions created by the bacteria in the biofilm are not easily opsonized and block signaling in polymorph nuclear leukocytes [47–49]. Within the macrophage, *Mycobacterium tuberculosis* to evade fusion with the lysosome requires eukaryotic serine/threonine protein kinase G (PKG). Protein kinase G can accelerate hydrolysis of NADH or FAD to maintain an optimum redox potential in macrophage. They also associated with *mycobacterial* nudix hydroxylase (RenU) [50–52]. Disruption or degradation of the PKG-RenU pathway disrupts mycobacterial biofilm growth, *mycobacteria* susceptibility to oxidative stress, and disrupts biofilm growth, and reduces TB survival in macrophages [51, 53]. Studies have shown that the DNA of *Mycobacterium tuberculosis* from cells such as macrophages isolate and reproduce in this cell [54, 55]. Survival of *Mycobacterium tuberculosis* (MTB) in macrophages plays a very important role in bacterial pathogenesis in the host. But the important point is that life inside the macrophage is not the only determinant of pathogenesis, and the bacterium is able to bind and infect more diverse cells, including alveolar and interstitial macrophages, type II pneumocytes, endothelial cells, and fibroblasts [54]. The biofilms evaded TLR2 and TLR9 which are bacterial recognition receptors used by macrophages. Host inflammatory responses such as TNF-α, IL-1β, and several others were found to be attenuated. The levels of iNOS, responsible for synthesizing reactive nitrogen intermediates that have microbicidal activities, were observed to be significantly reduced. A corresponding increase in arginase-1 expression levels was observed. All that has been said and what humans have so far failed to identify is a plausible explanation for the persistence of biofilm in vivo. Given that *Mycobacterium tuberculosis* is capable of proliferating in a variety of cells, biofilm formation, and infection can play a critical role in the severity of the disease, the complexity of treatment, the development of multidrug resistance, and many others [56–59]. Wolff et al. found in their study that in *mycobacteria* both biofilm growth and host persistence were regulated by through the PknG-modulated RHOCS, a newly identified hemostatic redox system in which PknG plays a key role [51].

2.2 Efflux pumps

The bacterial efflux pump family is divided into at least six groups which are mainly chromosomal: ABC,[6] SMR,[7] MFS,[8] MATE,[9] PACE,[10] RND.[11] The bacterial efflux pump family has several members including MexAB-OprM,[12] MexCD-OprJ, MexEF-OprN and MexXY-OprM, and MexAB-OprM, all of which are part of the RND family. The efflux pump can cause the transfer of internal or imported substances from the bacterial cytoplasm and its transfer to another environment, or limit the permeability of the outer membrane and purine and prevent drug access to the target [60–62]. Differences in physicochemical characteristics, molecular interactions, and protein binding sites are effective in choosing the substrate of efflux pumps and can cover a wide range or only for a specific substrate some of the main substrates of efflux pumps are antibiotics, disinfectants, aromatic hydrocarbons, antiseptics, and anti-virulence compounds and etc. [63–66].

3. Strategy to treatment

3.1 Antimicrobial peptides (AMPs)

Resistance to several drugs has increased as a result of excessive use of antibiotics both in medicine and in the field of livestock and poultry and has turned it into one of the most important problems today in various fields of medicine, especially healthcare. Antimicrobial peptides (AMPs) fight microbes with unique mechanisms and destroy them through different methods, which has led to extensive research in

---

[6] The ATP-binding cassette.

[7] The small multidrug resistance.

[8] The major facilitator superfamily.

[9] The multidrug and toxic compound extrusion.

[10] The proteobacterial antimicrobial compound efflux.

[11] The resistance/nodulation/cell division.

[12] A multidrug efflux protein expressed in the Gram-negative Pseudomonas aeruginosa.

this field and proposed them as an alternative to antibiotics. AMPs have the property of targeting different parts of microorganisms such as DNA, RNA, protein synthesis and folding, and inhibition of cellular life activities such as normal metabolism or cell division (**Table 1**) [12, 67]. Peptides are amphiphiles that interact with the surface of the bacterial cell with a negative charge and eventually cause the destruction of the cell membrane and the death of the bacteria. AMPs can inhibit basic processes in cells such as nucleic acid synthesis, protein biosynthesis, and cell wall biosynthesis. AMPs such as DM3, CP 10A, Microcin j25, and HNP-1 are effective on RNA. DM3, CP 10A Ostricacin-1, Ostricacin-2, PR-39, Indolicidin, Oabac5mini, Tachyplesin are effective on DNA. Apidaecin Hb1a peptides, Bac7 1-35, DM3 act on the ribosome. Magainin 1, Pleurocidin, CP10A, PR-39, and HNP-1 peptides are effective in protein biosynthesis and metabolism, and Indolicidin and Diptericin peptides are effective in cell division.

Cellular targets	AMPs
DNA	HNP-1 Buforin п BF2-A Indolicidin Oabac5mini Tachyplesin
RNA	DM3 Buforin пHNP-1 CP 10 AMicrocin j25 BF2-C
Ribosome	DM3 Bac7 1-35 Apidaecin Hb1a
Protein biosynthesis and metabolism	CP10A Pleurocidin PR-39 HNP-1 DM3 Magainin 1
Chaperone	Pyrrhocoricin Bac7 1-35 Drosocin Abaecin Oncocin Ixodidin ApidaecinHb 1a
Cell wall biosynthesis	Mersacidin Nisin Plectasin
Cell division	PR-39 Diptericin Microcin J25 Indolicidin HD5PR-26

Table 1.
Some of cellular targets of AMPs [12].

Some peptides have entered the clinical trials phase as a treatment for diseases, such as peptid LL-37 in Chronic leg ulcers, Melanoma, peptide NP213 in Onychomycosis, peptide AP 138 in MRSA implant infections, peptide HB 1345 in Acne, Trichophyton infections, peptide OG-716 in Clostridium difficile infections [68]. Polymer mimics of AMPs, peptidomimetic, or small-size oligomers are approaches that have proposed the idea of designing molecules Synthetic Mimics of Antimicrobial Peptides (SMAMPs). Due to the problems of protease instability, toxicity, and high cost of making AMPs, this idea has been discussed more than before [69]. AMPs are one of the most important lines of defense of organisms and often protect them against microbial pathogens. Cationic and non-cationic peptides are found in various organisms including bacteria and can act synergistically to improve immune responses to infections. They have multifunctional effects on innate immunity and provide antimicrobial activity against a wide range of microorganisms.

3.2 Nanoparticle

Nanoparticles (NPs) are small materials with a size of less than 100 nm, which is the reason for their physicochemical properties, including electrical and thermal conductivity, melting point, wettability, catalytic activity, light absorption, and scattering. It is widely used in the active field of research, economics, and also in the fields of intermediate applications, including for the purpose of therapeutic use in medical fields [70]. Nanoparticles have a small size and can be compared to virus particles such as human immunodeficiency virus (HIV) which are about 100 nanometers. NP can enter the blood through different routes such as the skin or inhalation and through it reach different parts of the body such as the liver, heart, or blood cells [71]. Inorganic nanomaterials such as gold, silver with the help of nanotechnology have promising applications in diagnosis, biomarkers, treatment of various types of diseases, biological imaging, and many other cases [72]. Silver nanoparticles (AgNPs) have antimicrobial potential, by making changes and modifications in them with the help of nanotechnology and their own physicochemical properties, it can be made more targeted against microbial agents. The biocompatibility, surface performance, and optical properties of gold nanoparticles (AuNPs) have caused the antibacterial effects of these nanoparticles (**Table 2**). Studies have shown the effect of nanoparticles against MDR bacteria such as *Escherichia coli* and *Streptococcus pyogenes* erythromycin-resistant, methicillin-resistant *Staphylococcus aureus* (MRSA) and ampicillin-resistant *Pseudomonas aeruginosa* [96, 97].

3.3 Bacteriophage therapy

In 1915, Frederick William Twort identified phages as potentially important antibacterial agents. Bacteriophages are those viruses that act specifically to infect bacteria and use special receptors for the interaction between themselves and the bacteria. The non-observation of resistant cases and their natural feature in destroying bacteria has raised bacteriophages or phages as a new and alternative treatment method in the future against bacterial infections [68, 98]. The discovery of antibiotics (initially with penicillin) created a revolution in dealing with pathogenic agents, and other treatments received less attention. Among the advantages of bacteriophage therapy, due to its self-propagating nature, a low dose can be administered (i.e., a small number of phages allows the production of more particles at the site of infection) [99, 100]. In addition to the many advantages of bacteriophage therapy, it also

No	Nanoparticles	Target microorganisms	References
1	Silver nanoparticles	*Escherichia Coli, Pseudomonas aeruginosa, Bacillus subtilis, Vibrio cholerae, Salmonella typhus Staphylococcus Aureus, Staphylococcus epidermidis, Phoma glomerata, Phoma herbarum, Fusarium semitectum, Trichoderma sp. and Candida albicans*	[73–75]
2	Silver ions	*Staphylococcus aureus and Escherichia coli, Pseudomonas aeruginosa*	[76, 77]
3	Silver zeolite	*Staphylococcus aureus, Escherichia coli*	[78]
4	Silver nitrate	*Escherichia coli, Pseudomonas aeruginosa, and Staphylococcus aureus, Proteus species, Periodontal pathogens*	[76, 79]
5	Silver ions	*Escherichia coli, Staphylococcus aureus, RNA viruses*	[80, 81]
6	Silver nanoparticles coated medical devices,	*Staphylococcus aureus and Streptococcus mutans,*	[82]
7	Bacterial cellulose-silver nanoparticles composite	*Escherichia coli and Staphylococcus aureus*	[83]
8	Silver nanoparticles impregnated on the wound dressing	*Pseudomonas aeruginosa, and Acinetobacter baumannii, Escherichia coli and Staphylococcus aureus, Proteus mirabilis, Candida albicans*	[84, 85]
9	Silver nanoparticles on cotton Fabrics	*Staphylococcus aureus, Escherichia coli*	[86]
10	TiO2Nps	*Staphylococcus. aureus, Escherichia coli, Bacillus. cereus*	[87, 88]
11	MgONps	*Escherichia. coli, Streptococcus mutants, Proteus vulgaris, Bacillus, Staphylococcus aureus*	[89, 90]
12	ZnONps	*Bacillus cereus, Staphylococcus. aureus, Escherichia coli, Klebsiella pneumonia, and salmonella typhi, Bacillus cereus*	[91–93]
13	CuONps	*Klebsiella, Escherichia coli, Staphylococcus. aureus, Bacillus. subtili,*	[94, 95]

Table 2.
Activity of nanoparticles against broad spectrum of microorganisms.

has limitations, among which the following can be mentioned: the need for specific protein receptors on the surface of bacteria, the limitation of their number as a target (which means that to fight against one type of bacteria, several different phages is needed) and Lack of pharmacokinetic properties [68, 101]. There are different types of bacteriophages, and lytic phages are the most common treatment methods that contribute to the death of bacteria by inducing cell lysis. In the treatment of bacteriophage using lytic phage, the connection to the outer membrane of bacterial cells is done first, and the genetic material is transferred. Phage-specific enzymes are secreted after the interaction between tail strands and host cell surface receptors and can destroy different parts of bacteria, including lipopolysaccharide and peptidoglycan (in Gram-negative bacteria, outer membrane). After that, the gene is expressed, the phage DNA is amplified and the host cell is controlled [99]. Many research groups conducted studies aimed at bacteriophage treatment, but more extensive studies are needed for clinical use. In a study that aimed to treat bacteriophage (P2, 3/113) with trial number NCT03140085, the use of bacteriophages against antibiotic resistance pathogens in the treatment of urinary tract infections was investigated, in another study of bacteriophage therapy for the treatment of leg ulcers. Non-infectious and infected diabetics with *P. aeruginosa*, *Staphylococcus aureus,* and/or *Acinetobacter baumanni* were used. In a study conducted by Leitner L et al., Bacteriophage has been used to treat *Pseudomonas. aeruginosa* cystic fibrosis. Many research groups conducted studies aimed at bacteriophage treatment, but more extensive studies are needed for clinical use. In a study that aimed to treat bacteriophage (P2, 3/113) with trial number NCT03140085, the use of bacteriophages against antibiotic resistance pathogens in the treatment of urinary tract infections was investigated [102], In another study Kothari et al. in 2023 were used bacteriophage therapy for the treatment of leg ulcers, Non-infectious and infected diabetics with *Pseudomonas. aeruginosa*, *Staphylococcus aureus* and/or *Acinetobacter baumanni* [103]. In the study of Hraiech et al., bacteriophage was used to treat cystic fibrosis of *Pseudomonas. aeruginosa* [104]. Although studies have shown resistance to phage in clinical trials, the rate of resistance in them is much lower than that of antibiotics, but despite this, more studies are needed to evaluate the exact performance of bacteriophage in treatment [105].

4. Conclusions

The increasing and indiscriminate use of antibiotics has turned drug resistance into one of the main problems facing the health of societies. Bacterial adaptation and, on the other hand, intrinsic and acquired resistance of bacteria have contributed to the spread of MDR/XDR infections caused by microorganisms. However, finding a suitable treatment approach to prevent and stop the process of antibiotic resistance seems necessary. The process of biofilm formation and efflux pumps is one of the effective mechanisms for creating and increasing the resistance mechanism in bacteria. It has been shown that the use of antimicrobial peptides, nanoparticle, phage therapy, and some new generation antibiotics are suitable candidates for new treatment strategy as an alternative to conventional treatment considering these future treatments should be more targeted and prioritize new treatments in order to reduce the spread of antibiotic resistance.

Acknowledgements

The authors would like to thank all those who provided expert technical assistance.

Conflicts of interest

The authors declare no conflict of interest.

Author details

Saeid Besharati[1,2]

1 Nursing Research Center of Respiratory Diseases (NRCRD), National Research Institute of Tuberculosis and Lung Diseases (NRITLD), Shahid Beheshti University of Medicine Science, Tehran, Iran

2 Department of Microbiology and Microbial Biotechnology, Faculty of Life Sciences and Biotechnology, Shahid Beheshti University, Iran

*Address all correspondence to: saeid.besharati@gmail.com

References

[1] Salam MA, Al-Amin MY, Salam MT, Pawar JS, Akhter N, Rabaan AA, et al. Antimicrobial resistance: A growing serious threat for global public health. Healthcare. MDPI; 2023;**11**(13):1946

[2] Shallcross LJ, Howard SJ, Fowler T, Davies SC. Tackling the threat of antimicrobial resistance: From policy to sustainable action. Philosophical Transactions of the Royal Society B: Biological Sciences. 2015;**370**(1670):20140082. DOI: 10.1098/rstb.2014.0082

[3] O'Neill J. Tackling Drug-Resistant Infections Globally: Final Report and Recommendations. Government of the United Kingdom; 2016. Landmark report that analysed the impact of antimicrobial resistance from an economic perspective, which is the source of the highly quoted figure that antimicrobial resistance will cause. 2022;10

[4] Villa TG, Feijoo-Siota L, Sánchez-Pérez A, Rama JR, Sieiro C. Horizontal gene transfer in bacteria, an overview of the mechanisms involved. Horizontal Gene. Cham, Switzerland, New York, NY, USA: Springer; 2019. pp. 3-76

[5] Gogarten JP, Townsend JP. Horizontal gene transfer, genome innovation and evolution. Nature Reviews Microbiology. 2005;**3**(9):679-687

[6] Gaurav A, Bakht P, Saini M, Pandey S, Pathania R. Role of bacterial efflux pumps in antibiotic resistance, virulence, and strategies to discover novel efflux pump inhibitors. Microbiology. 2023;**169**(5):001333

[7] Besharati S, Owlia P, Sadeghi A, Ahmadi F, Fani F, Puladfar G, et al. Frequency, antibiotic resistance, and serogroups of salmonella among chicken meat specimens in Tehran, Iran. Daneshvar Medicine. 2020;**27**(4):1-10

[8] Arabshahi A, Ariyanfar M. Health tourism and medical tourism capabilities in Iran. Geographical Journal of Tourism Space. 2014;**3**(9):133-152

[9] Besharati S, Sadeghi A, Ahmadi F, Tajeddin E, Salehi RM, Fani F, et al. Serogroups, and drug resistance of nontyphoidal salmonella in symptomatic patients with community-acquired diarrhea and chicken meat samples in Tehran. Iranian Journal of Veterinary Research. 2020;**21**(4):269

[10] Von Wintersdorff CJ, Penders J, Van Niekerk JM, Mills ND, Majumder S, Van Alphen LB, et al. Dissemination of antimicrobial resistance in microbial ecosystems through horizontal gene transfer. Frontiers in Microbiology. 2016;7:173

[11] Lachaud L, Fernández-Arévalo A, Normand A-C, Lami P, Nabet C, Donnadieu JL, et al. Identification of leishmania by matrix-assisted laser desorption ionization–time of flight (MALDI-TOF) mass spectrometry using a free web-based application and a dedicated mass-spectral library. Journal of Clinical Microbiology. 2017;**55**(10):2924-2933

[12] Moradi M, Besharati S, Moghaddam MM, Fasihi-Ramandi M, Azad ZM, Mirnejad R. A concise review on the antimicrobial peptides and their critical activity against intracellular targets of bacteria. Journal of Microbiology, Biotechnology and Food Sciences. 2023;**12**(4):e6006-e

[13] Farnia P, Besharati S, Farina P, Ayoubi S, Marjani M, Ghanavi J, et al. The role of efflux pumps transporter in multi-drug resistant tuberculosis: Mycobacterial memberane protein (MmpL5). The International Journal of Mycobacteriology. 2024;**13**(1):7-14

[14] Besharati S, Owlia P, Sadeghi A, Ahmadi F, Alebouyeh M. Frequency of integrons 1 and 2 and their relationship with drug resistance patterns of salmonella isolates in patients with gastroenteritis in Tehran, Iran. Daneshvar Medicine. 2020;**28**(5):1-10

[15] Lehtinen S, Blanquart F, Lipsitch M, Fraser C, Collaboration wtMP. On the evolutionary ecology of multidrug resistance in bacteria. PLoS Pathogens. 2019;**15**(5):e1007763

[16] Jamal M, Ahmad W, Andleeb S, Jalil F, Imran M, Nawaz MA, et al. Bacterial biofilm and associated infections. Journal of the Chinese Medical Association. 2018;**81**(1):7-11

[17] Fouladi MD, Besharati S, Farnia P, Khosravi A. A concise review of the effect of efflux pump on biofilm intensity in bacteria with a special view to mycobacterium. Journal of Preventive, Diagnostic and Treatment Strategies in Medicine. 2024;**3**(1):1-5

[18] Besharati S, Farnia P, Farnia P, Ghanavi J, Velayati AA. Investigation of the hypothesis of biofilm formation in coronavirus (COVID-19). Biomedical and Biotechnology Research Journal (BBRJ). 2020;**4**(Suppl 1):S99-S100

[19] Besharati S, Owlia P. Evaluation of biofilm production capacity in salmonella isolated from chicken meat in Tehran municipally daily fruit and vegetable markets. Daneshvar Medicine. 2020;**28**(1):62-72

[20] Davarzani F, Saidi N, Besharati S, Saderi H, Rasooli I, Owlia P. Evaluation of antibiotic resistance pattern, alginate and biofilm production in clinical isolates of *Pseudomonas aeruginosa*. Iranian Journal of Public Health. 2021;**50**(2):341

[21] Flemming H-C, Wingender J, Szewzyk U, Steinberg P, Rice SA, Kjelleberg S. Biofilms: An emergent form of bacterial life. Nature Reviews Microbiology. 2016;**14**(9):563-575

[22] Halan B, Buehler K, Schmid A. Biofilms as living catalysts in continuous chemical syntheses. Trends in Biotechnology. 2012;**30**(9):453-465

[23] Polyudova TV, Eroshenko DV, Pimenova EV. The biofilm formation of nontuberculous mycobacteria and its inhibition by essential oils. The International Journal of Mycobacteriology. 2021;**10**(1):43-50

[24] Lewis AH, Falkinham JO III. Microaerobic growth and anaerobic survival of *Mycobacterium avium*, *Mycobacterium intracellulare* and *Mycobacterium scrofulaceum*. International Journal of Mycobacteriology. 2015;**4**(1):25-30

[25] Batoni G, Maisetta G, Esin S. Antimicrobial peptides and their interaction with biofilms of medically relevant bacteria. Biochimica et Biophysica Acta (BBA)-Biomembranes. 2016;**1858**(5):1044-1060

[26] Cieplik F, Deng D, Crielaard W, Buchalla W, Hellwig E, Al-Ahmad A, et al. Antimicrobial photodynamic therapy–what we know and what we don't. Critical Reviews in Microbiology. 2018;**44**(5):571-589

[27] Govaert M, Smet C, Vergauwen L, Ećimović B, Walsh JL, Baka M, et al. Influence of plasma characteristics

on the efficacy of cold atmospheric plasma (CAP) for inactivation of listeria monocytogenes and *Salmonella typhimurium* biofilms. Innovative Food Science and Emerging Technologies. 2019;**52**:376-386

[28] Pletzer D, Coleman SR, Hancock RE. Anti-biofilm peptides as a new weapon in antimicrobial warfare. Current Opinion in Microbiology. 2016;**33**:35-40

[29] Mehrishi P, Agarwal P, Broor S, Sharma A. Antibacterial and antibiofilm properties of *Azadirachta indica* (neem), *Aloe vera* (Aloe vera), and *Mentha piperita* (peppermint) against multidrug-resistant clinical isolates. Biomedical and Biotechnology Research Journal. 2022;**6**:98-104

[30] Alizadeh M, Vasebi Y, Safaie N. Microbial antagonists against plant pathogens in Iran: A review. Open Agriculture. 2020;**5**(1):404-440

[31] Bjarnsholt T, Alhede M, Alhede M, Eickhardt-Sørensen SR, Moser C, Kühl M, et al. The in vivo biofilm. Trends in Microbiology. 2013;**21**(9):466-474

[32] Deysine M. Infections associated with surgical implants. The New England Journal of Medicine. 2004;**351**(2):193-195

[33] Goswami M. Antibacterial activity of some medicinal plants and antibiotics against *Staphylococcus aureus* and *Mammaliicoccus sciuri* isolated from acne. Biomedical and Biotechnology Research Journal (BBRJ). 1 Jul 2022;**6**(3):372-381

[34] Del Pozo JL. Biofilm-related disease. Expert Review of Anti-Infective Therapy. 2018;**16**(1):51-65

[35] Donlan RM, Costerton JW. Biofilms: Survival mechanisms of clinically relevant microorganisms. Clinical Microbiology Reviews. 2002;**15**(2):167-193

[36] Malik S, Rana JS, Nehra K. Prevalence and antibiotic susceptibility pattern of uropathogenic *Escherichia Coli* strains in Sonipat region of Haryana in India. Biomedical and Biotechnology Research Journal (BBRJ). 2021;**5**(1):80

[37] Bedi B, Maurice NM, Sadikot RT. Microarchitecture of Pseudomonas aeruginosa biofilms: A biological perspective. Biomedical and Biotechnology Research Journal (BBRJ). 2018;**2**(4):227-236

[38] Chung PY, Khanum R. Antimicrobial peptides as potential anti-biofilm agents against multidrug-resistant bacteria. Journal of Microbiology, Immunology, and Infection. 2017;**50**(4):405-410

[39] Gondil VS, Chhibber S. Exploring potential of phage therapy for tuberculosis using model organism. Biomedical and Biotechnology Research Journal (BBRJ). 2018;**2**(1):9

[40] Xu M, Hu Y, Xiao Y, Zhang Y, Sun K, Wu T, et al. Near-infrared-controlled nanoplatform exploiting photothermal promotion of peroxidase-like and OXD-like activities for potent antibacterial and anti-biofilm therapies. ACS Applied Materials and Interfaces. 2020;**12**(45):50260-50274

[41] Amini M, Ghanavi J, Farnia P, Karimi M, Ghomi H. In vitro antiproliferative activity of cold atmospheric plasma on small-cell lung carcinoma. Biomedical and Biotechnology Research Journal (BBRJ). 2020;**4**(1):76

[42] Allaker RP, Memarzadeh K. Nanoparticles and the control of oral

infections. International Journal of Antimicrobial Agents. 2014;**43**(2):95-104

[43] Besinis A, De Peralta T, Tredwin CJ, Handy RD. Review of nanomaterials in dentistry: Interactions with the oral microenvironment, clinical applications, hazards, and benefits. ACS Nano. 2015;**9**(3):2255-2289

[44] Santhanam R, Weinhold A, Goldberg J, Oh Y, Baldwin IT. Native root-associated bacteria rescue a plant from a sudden-wilt disease that emerged during continuous cropping. National Academy of Sciences of the United States of America. 2015;**112**(36):E5013-E5E20

[45] Nagesh M, Asokan R, Mohan K. Partial characterization of novel nematicidal toxins from Bacillus cereus Frankland and Frankland 1887 and their effect on root-knot nematode, Meloidogyne incognita (Kofoid & White) Chitwood. Journal of Biological Control. 2005;**19**(1):65-70

[46] Ahmadi F, Sadeghi A, Besharati S, Saffarian P, Tajedini E, Owlia P, et al. Investigation of frequency and antimicrobial resistance patterns of Shiga toxigenic Escherichia coli in vegetable samples from Tehran, Iran. Iranian Journal of Nutrition Sciences and Food Technology. 2023;**18**(2):89-96

[47] Günther F, Wabnitz GH, Stroh P, Prior B, Obst U, Samstag Y, et al. Host defence against Staphylococcus aureus biofilms infection: Phagocytosis of biofilms by polymorphonuclear neutrophils (PMN). Molecular Immunology. 2009;**46**(8-9):1805-1813

[48] FazliM,BjarnsholtT,Kirketerp-MøllerK, Jørgensen B, Andersen AS, Krogfelt KA, et al.NonrandomdistributionofPseudomonas aeruginosa and Staphylococcus aureus in chronic wounds. Journal of Clinical Microbiology. 2009;**47**(12):4084-4089

[49] Farnia TP, Ghanavi J, Besharati S, Farnia P, Velayati AA. The pili at genomic level. Pili in mycobacterium tuberculosis: Structure, function, and therapeutic advances. Elsever eBook; 2024:161. ISBN: 9780443217135, Paperback ISBN: 9780443217128. Available from: https://shop.elsevier.com/books/pili-in-mycobacterium-tuberculosis/velayati/978-0-443-21712-8

[50] Armstrong J, Hart PDA. Response of cultured macrophages to mycobacterium tuberculosis, with observations on fusion of lysosomes with phagosomes. The Journal of Experimental Medicine. 1971;**134**(3):713-740

[51] Wolff KA, Nguyen HT, Cartabuke RH, Singh A, Ogwang S, Nguyen L. Protein kinase G is required for intrinsic antibiotic resistance in mycobacteria. Antimicrob Agents Chemother. Aug 2009;**53**(8):3515-3519. DOI: 10.1128/AAC.00012-09. Epub 2009 Jun 15

[52] Varahram M, Besharati S, Farnia P, Ghanavi J, Saif S, Nia JH, et al. Correlation of single-nucleotide polymorphism at interferon-gamma R1 (at position- 56) in positive purified protein derivative health workers with COVID-19 infection. The International Journal of Mycobacteriology. 2022;**11**(3):318-322

[53] Besharati S, Aghajani J, Farnia P, Ayoubi S, Kalantari L, Farnia P, Ghanavi J, et al. Association between the Vitamin D Receptor Gene (FokI, BsmI, ApaI, and TaqI) Polymorphism in Health-care Workers and Susceptibility to COVID-19. Biomedical and Biotechnology Research Journal (BBRJ). 1 Jul 2023;**7**(3):404-410

[54] Hernandez-Pando R, Jeyanathan M, Mengistu G, Aguilar D, Orozco H, Harboe M, et al. Persistence of DNA

from mycobacterium tuberculosis in superficially normal lung tissue during latent infection. The Lancet. 2000;**356**(9248):2133-2138

[55] Russell DG. Mycobacterium tuberculosis: Here today, and here tomorrow. Nature Reviews Molecular Cell Biology. 2001;**2**(8):569-578

[56] Rabin N, Zheng Y, Opoku-Temeng C, Du Y, Bonsu E, Sintim HO. Biofilm formation mechanisms and targets for developing antibiofilm agents. Future Medicinal Chemistry. 2015;**7**(4):493-512

[57] Landini P, Antoniani D, Burgess JG, Nijland R. Molecular mechanisms of compounds affecting bacterial biofilm formation and dispersal. Applied Microbiology and Biotechnology. 2010;**86**(3):813-823

[58] Farnia TP, Farnia P, Besharati S, Ghanavi J, Velayati AA. Role of mycobacterium tuberculosis pili in host. Pili in mycobacterium tuberculosis: Structure, function, and therapeutic advances. Elsever eBook; 2024:263. Available from: https://shop.elsevier.com/books/pili-in-mycobacterium-tuberculosis/velayati/978-0-443-21712-8. Paperback ISBN: 9780443217128 eBook ISBN: 9780443217135

[59] Farnia P, Farnia P, Ghanavi J, Ayoubi S, Besharati S, Velayati AA. Comparison of proline-glutamate-proline-glutamate-polymorphic GC-rich sequences family protein Wag22 (Rv1759c), PE_PGRS31 (Rv1768), PE_PGRS32 (Rv1803), and PE_PGRS33 gene (Rv1818c) in exponential state and under in vitro model of latency in same clinical isolates of mycobacterium tuberculosis: Frameshift mutation in extensively drug-resistant and totally drug-resistant tuberculosis bacilli. Biomedical and Biotechnology Research Journal (BBRJ). 2023;7(4):621-632

[60] Piddock LJ. Multidrug-resistance efflux pumps? Not just for resistance. Nature Reviews Microbiology. 2006;**4**(8):629-636

[61] Sun J, Deng Z, Yan A. Bacterial multidrug efflux pumps: Mechanisms, physiology and pharmacological exploitations. Biochemical and Biophysical Research Communications. 2014;**453**(2):254-267

[62] Hassan KA, Liu Q, Elbourne LD, Ahmad I, Sharples D, Naidu V, et al. Pacing across the membrane: The novel PACE family of efflux pumps is widespread in gram-negative pathogens. Research in Microbiology. 2018;**169**(7-8):450-454

[63] Zwama M, Yamaguchi A, Nishino K. Phylogenetic and functional characterisation of the haemophilus influenzae multidrug efflux pump AcrB. Communications Biology. 2019;**2**(1):340

[64] Mehla J, Malloci G, Mansbach R, López CA, Tsivkovski R, Haynes K, et al. Predictive rules of efflux inhibition and avoidance in *Pseudomonas aeruginosa*. MBio. 23 Feb 2021;**12**(1):10-128

[65] Nishino K, Yamaguchi A. Analysis of a complete library of putative drug transporter genes in *Escherichia coli*. Journal of Bacteriology. 2001;**183**(20):5803-5812

[66] Sanz-García F, Gil-Gil T, Laborda P, Ochoa-Sánchez LE, Martínez JL, Hernando-Amado S. Coming from the wild: Multidrug resistant opportunistic pathogens presenting a primary, not human-linked, environmental habitat. International Journal of Molecular Sciences. 2021;**22**(15):8080

[67] Browne K, Chakraborty S, Chen R, Willcox MD, Black DS, Walsh WR, et al. A new era of antibiotics: The clinical potential of antimicrobial peptides.

International Journal of Molecular Sciences. 2020;**21**(19):7047

[68] Ghosh C, Sarkar P, Issa R, Haldar J. Alternatives to conventional antibiotics in the era of antimicrobial resistance. Trends in Microbiology. 2019;**27**(4):323-338

[69] Scorciapino MA, Rinaldi AC. Antimicrobial peptidomimetics: Reinterpreting nature to deliver innovative therapeutics. Frontiers in Immunology. 2012;**3**:171

[70] Jeevanandam J, Barhoum A, Chan YS, Dufresne A, Danquah MK. Review on nanoparticles and nanostructured materials: History, sources, toxicity and regulations. Beilstein Journal of Nanotechnology. 2018;**9**(1):1050-1074

[71] Buzea C, Pacheco II, Robbie K. Nanomaterials and nanoparticles: Sources and toxicity. Biointerphases. 2007;**2**(4):MR17-MR71

[72] Singh R, Nalwa HS. Medical applications of nanoparticles in biological imaging, cell labeling, antimicrobial agents, and anticancer nanodrugs. Journal of Biomedical Nanotechnology. 2011;**7**(4):489-503

[73] Escárcega-González CE, Garza-Cervantes JA, Vazquez-Rodríguez A, Montelongo-Peralta LZ, Treviño-Gonzalez MT, Díaz Barriga Castro E, et al. In vivo antimicrobial activity of silver nanoparticles produced via a green chemistry synthesis using Acacia rigidula as a reducing and capping agent. International Journal of Nanomedicine. 2018:2349-2363

[74] Gajbhiye M, Kesharwani J, Ingle A, Gade A, Rai M. Fungus-mediated synthesis of silver nanoparticles and their activity against pathogenic fungi in combination with fluconazole. Nanomedicine: Nanotechnology, Biology and Medicine. 2009;**5**(4):382-386

[75] Ingle A, Gade A, Pierrat S, Sonnichsen C, Rai M. Mycosynthesis of silver nanoparticles using the fungus Fusarium acuminatum and its activity against some human pathogenic bacteria. Current Nanoscience. 2008;**4**(2):141-144

[76] Pormohammad A, Turner RJ. Silver antibacterial synergism activities with eight other metal (loid)-based antimicrobials against Escherichia coli, Pseudomonas aeruginosa, and Staphylococcus aureus. Antibiotics. 2020;**9**(12):853

[77] Feng QL, Wu J, Chen G-Q, Cui F-Z, Kim T, Kim J. A mechanistic study of the antibacterial effect of silver ions on Escherichia coli and Staphylococcus aureus. Journal of Biomedical Materials Research. 2000;**52**(4):662-668

[78] Dutta P, Wang B. Zeolite-supported silver as antimicrobial agents. Coordination Chemistry Reviews. 2019;**383**:1-29

[79] Richards RME, Taylor RB, Xing DK. An evaluation of the antibacterial activities of combinations of sulfonamides, trimethoprim, dibromopropamidine, and silver nitrate compared with their uptakes by selected bacteria. Journal of Pharmaceutical Sciences. 1991;**80**(9):861-867

[80] Xu Z, Zhang C, Wang X, Liu D. Release strategies of silver ions from materials for bacterial killing. ACS Applied Bio Materials. 2021;**4**(5):3985-3999

[81] Thurman RB, Gerba CP, Bitton G. The molecular mechanisms of copper and silver ion disinfection of bacteria

and viruses. Critical Reviews in Environmental Science and Technology. 1989;**18**(4):295-315

[82] Yin IX, Zhang J, Zhao IS, Mei ML, Li Q, Chu CH. The antibacterial mechanism of silver nanoparticles and its application in dentistry. International Journal of Nanomedicine. 2020:2555-2562

[83] Barud HS, Regiani T, Marques RF, Lustri WR, Messaddeq Y, Ribeiro SJ. Antimicrobial bacterial cellulose-silver nanoparticles composite membranes. Journal of Nanomaterials. 2011;**2011**(1):721631

[84] Dahm H. Silver nanoparticles in wound infections: Present status and future prospects. In: Nanotechnology in Skin, Soft Tissue, and Bone Infections. 2020. pp. 151-168

[85] Vivcharenko V, Trzaskowska M, Przekora A. Wound dressing modifications for accelerated healing of infected wounds. International Journal of Molecular Sciences. 2023;**24**(8):7193

[86] Shilpa SA, Subbulakshmi M, Hikku G. Nanoparticles of metal/metal oxide embedded fabrics to impart antibacterial activity to counteract hospital acquired infections. Engineering Research Express. 2022;**4**(3):032002

[87] Sharma P, Kumari R, Yadav M, Lal R. Evaluation of TiO2 nanoparticles physicochemical parameters associated with their antimicrobial applications. Indian Journal of Microbiology. 2022;**62**(3):338-350

[88] Landage KS, Arbade GK, Khanna P, Bhongale CJ. Biological approach to synthesize TiO2 nanoparticles using Staphylococcus aureus for antibacterial and anti-biofilm applications. Journal of Microbiology & Experimentation. 2020;**8**(1):36-43

[89] Sharma N, Jandaik S, Singh TG, Kumar S. Nanoparticles: Boon to mankind and bane to pathogens. In: Nanobiomaterials in Antimicrobial Therapy. 2016. pp. 483-509

[90] Chattopadhyay I. Application of nanoparticles in drug delivery. In: Model Organisms to Study Biological Activities and Toxicity of Nanoparticles. 2020. pp. 35-57

[91] Kudaer N, Risan MH, Yousif E, Kadhom M, Raheem R, Hairunisa N, et al. Effect of ZnO nanoparticles as antimicrobial on multidrug resistance Klebsiella pneumonia: A review. Jurnal Biomedika dan Kesehatan. 2022;**5**(3):236-242

[92] Umar H, Kavaz D, Rizaner N. Biosynthesis of zinc oxide nanoparticles using Albizia lebbeck stem bark, and evaluation of its antimicrobial, antioxidant, and cytotoxic activities on human breast cancer cell lines. International Journal of Nanomedicine. 2019:87-100

[93] Kalpana V, Devi RV. A review on green synthesis, biomedical applications, and toxicity studies of ZnO NPs. Bioinorganic Chemistry and Applications. 2018;**2018**(1):3569758

[94] Bhuvaneshwari V, Ramasamy NK, Kumar SI, Kalaivani S, Vaidehi D, Kumar DK. Antimicrobial activity of copper nanomaterials: Current status and future perspectives. In: Copper Nanostructures: Next-Generation of Agrochemicals for Sustainable Agroecosystems. 2022. pp. 453-475

[95] Alavi M, Moradi M. Different antibacterial and photocatalyst functions for herbal and bacterial synthesized

silver and copper/copper oxide nanoparticles/nanocomposites: A review. Inorganic Chemistry Communications. 2022;**142**:109590

[96] Rai MK, Deshmukh S, Ingle A, Gade A. Silver nanoparticles: The powerful nanoweapon against multidrug-resistant bacteria. Journal of Applied Microbiology. 2012;**112**(5):841-852

[97] Morones JR, Elechiguerra JL, Camacho A, Holt K, Kouri JB, Ramírez JT, et al. The bactericidal effect of silver nanoparticles. Nanotechnology. 2005;**16**(10):2346

[98] Lopetuso LR, Giorgio ME, Saviano A, Scaldaferri F, Gasbarrini A, Cammarota G. Bacteriocins and bacteriophages: Therapeutic weapons for gastrointestinal diseases? International Journal of Molecular Sciences. 2019;**20**(1):183

[99] Maciejewska B, Olszak T, Drulis-Kawa Z. Applications of bacteriophages versus phage enzymes to combat and cure bacterial infections: An ambitious and also a realistic application? Applied Microbiology and Biotechnology. 2018;**102**:2563-2581

[100] de Freitas Almeida GM, Sundberg L-R. The forgotten tale of Brazilian phage therapy. The Lancet Infectious Diseases. 2020;**20**(5):e90-e101

[101] Hyman P. Phages for phage therapy: Isolation, characterization, and host range breadth. Pharmaceuticals. 2019;**12**(1):35

[102] Leitner L, Sybesma W, Chanishvili N, Goderdzishvili M, Chkhotua A, Ujmajuridze A, et al. Bacteriophages for treating urinary tract infections in patients undergoing transurethral resection of the prostate: A randomized, placebo-controlled, double-blind clinical trial. BMC Urology. 2017;**17**:1-6

[103] Kothari A, Kherdekar R, Mago V, Uniyal M, Mamgain G, Kalia RB, et al. Age of antibiotic resistance in MDR/XDR clinical pathogen of *Pseudomonas aeruginosa*. Pharmaceuticals. 2023;**16**(9):1230

[104] Hraiech S, Brégeon F, Rolain J-M. Bacteriophage-based therapy in cystic fibrosis-associated *Pseudomonas aeruginosa* infections: Rationale and current status. Drug Design, Development and Therapy. 16 Jul 2015;**9**:3653-3663. DOI: 10.2147/DDDT.S53123

[105] Oechslin F. Resistance development to bacteriophages occurring during bacteriophage therapy. Viruses. 2018;**10**(7):351

Section 2

Innate Immunity and Cancer Therapy Challenges

Chapter 4

Neutropenia among Cancer Patients: Unravelling the Challenges and Complexities

Bassam Abdul Rasool Hassan and Ali Haider Mohammed

Abstract

Neutropenia, a deficiency in neutrophils (vital immune system cells), significantly compromises the body's ability to fight infections. In about 50% of cancer patients undergoing chemotherapy, especially in leukemia cases, neutropenia elevates the risk of severe, life-threatening infections due to inadequate neutrophil levels for combating pathogens. Prolonged or intense neutropenia episodes heighten infection susceptibility. Chemotherapy-induced neutropenia (CIN) can also cause lower chemotherapy doses and delays, which can make it harder to stick with treatment and could lower survival rates by making it harder to stick to chemotherapy schedules. CIN also adversely impacts the quality of life (QOL) and increases the risk of treatment failure. In addressing CIN, Chinese herbal medicine (CHM) has shown promising results in enhancing white blood cell counts as a supplementary treatment, outperforming conventional Western oral treatments in certain cases. However, managing neutropenia often involves an extensive use of broad-spectrum antibiotics, raising concerns over the emergence of multidrug-resistant bacteria strains. This underscores the importance of integrating antimicrobial stewardship programs into treatment protocols for cancer patients with neutropenia. The chapter delves into these aspects, exploring prevention and treatment strategies for neutropenia, particularly focusing on the implications of CIN.

Keywords: neutropenia, cancer disease, chemotherapy, negative impact, herbal treatment, antimicrobial stewardship

1. Introduction

Cancer has risen to prominence as one of the century's leading killers, second only to heart disease in terms of mortality rate. Chemotherapy is used to treat a wide variety of cancers, and a typical chemotherapy programme in the clinic involves the use of several different drugs [1–3].

Most of the people diagnosed with cancer will receive chemotherapy as part of their treatment plan. The medicines in these potent combination chemotherapy regimens are routinely given at the maximum safe doses. Over the course of months, patients undergo multiple cycles of chemotherapy, creating a highly toxic physiologic environment and increasing their risk for complications. Negative side effects from chemotherapy for cancer include neutropenia, anaemia, nausea and vomiting, mucositis, alopecia, pain, and fatigue. Hence, due to these reasons, cancer is considered as one of the major diseases that will negatively affect the quality of life [4–6].

There are various types of neutropenia, like congenital, cyclic, autoimmune, idiopathic, and chemotherapy-induced neutropenia, but the current chapter will focus on chemotherapy-induced neutropenia, i.e., the one caused by myelosuppressive chemotherapy.

1.1 Neutrophil cells

Neutrophil cells were first identified by Elie Metchnikoff [1] as an inflammatory immunological response triggered by the insertion of rose thorns into starfish larvae. Neutrophils make up between 45 and 70 per cent of all white blood cells (WBCs). Granules in neutrophils' cytoplasm include glycogen and antimicrobial compounds, earning them the names neutrophils, polymorphonuclear leucocytes, and granulocytes [2]. Haematopoietic stem cells in bone marrow synthesise and generate neutrophils. Maturation of neutrophils occurs after 10–14 days. Until the late 1990s, it was believed that neutrophils only lasted for 6–10 hours after being released into the bloodstream [2, 3]. Further, recent research has shown that neutrophils may facilitate the resolution of inflammation by producing anti-inflammatory chemicals [4]. In addition, research shows that neutrophils will phagocytose and remain active at the site of inflammation or infection for around 2–6 days [2, 4, 5].

1.2 Neutropenia

The medical condition known as neutropenia is characterised by a reduction in the total count of neutrophils present in the bloodstream. The clinical definition of neutropenia entails a reduction in the absolute neutrophil count (ANC) that exceeds two standard deviations below the established normal range. The patient is classified as neutropenic when their absolute neutrophil count (ANC) falls below the standard range of 1500 cells/μl or (1500 cells/mm^3) [4, 7].

About, febrile neutropenia (FN) (i.e., when the patient got a temperature) is most commonly linked to chemotherapy, it can also occur after irradiating the majority of the bone marrow. When neutropenia is present alongside a fever for more than an hour and the neutrophil count is less than 500 cells/μl or (500 cells/mm^3) or is expected to fall to less than 500 cells/μl or (500 cells/mm^3) within the next 48 hours, the condition is known as febrile neutropenia [8, 9].

2. Relationship between neutropenia and other toxicities

Most people diagnosed with cancer will receive chemotherapy as part of their treatment plan. The medicines in these potent combination chemotherapy regimens are routinely given at the maximum safe doses. Patients are exposed to a very toxic physiologic environment due to the multiple cycles of chemotherapy administered over the course of months [4, 5]. Neutropenia, anaemia, nausea, vomiting, mucositis, alopecia, discomfort, exhaustion, and soreness are only few of the usual side effects of cancer treatment were recorded, but the results were not statistically significant. In line with these results, a recent investigation discovered a link between the presence of FN and the presence of additional toxicities in grades 3 and 4. When preventative measures were implemented, the occurrence of the other negative impacts decreased. The quality of life of patients may be significantly impacted by the potential for unpleasant effects to become more severe in the presence of FN [4, 5].

3. Negative impact of neutropenia on chemotherapy treatment outcome

The evaluation of the treatment's effects on a patient's quality of life (QOL) is a natural next step after analysing the constellation of adverse effects of cancer chemotherapy. Neutropenia caused by chemotherapy and decreased QOL both have the potential to compromise the success of cancer treatment. Neutropenia is an objective indicator of poor treatment compliance because of the widespread use of dosage reductions and delays in response to chemotherapy-induced neutropenia (CIN). In addition, studies have shown that in some types of cancer, survival is correlated with adherence to the treatment schedule, which maintains the dose intensity of the chemotherapy. As a result, having CIN may lessen the effectiveness of treatment [4–6].

It appears that treatment outcomes are also affected by QOL deficits. Patients' motivation to continue chemotherapy can be significantly impacted by their QOL throughout treatment. Pretreatment quality of life has also been found to connect with survival. Patients with breast cancer, lung cancer, melanoma, and other malignancies have been studied, and the results show that a greater QOL before treatment is a significant predictor of survival. The quality of life of a patient improves throughout treatment, which is an independent prognostic factor. These findings demonstrate that CIN and QOL are two distinct factors that influence patient outcomes [4–6].

4. Negative impact of neutropenia on cancer patients QOL

Since CIN and decreased QOL each have their own detrimental effects on outcomes, it makes sense to examine how they are related to one another. For instance, does having CIN itself negatively impact QOL, hence increasing the likelihood of unsuccessful treatment? One could assume that the presence of CIN has a detrimental impact on QOL after reading about the methods for controlling neutropenia. Neutropenia's impact on QOL in cancer patients has been the subject of several recent research. In a prospective study of 62 patients undergoing treatment for a wide range of cancers, researchers found that 50% of patients experienced grade 4 neutropenia and that a greater decline in the ANC was associated with lower QOL at the time of the ANC nadir in the social functioning, distress, despair, and general physical symptoms subscales of the Psychosocial Adjustment to Illness Scale. Patients with grade 4 CIN also showed larger improvements in physical functioning, bodily pain, and general physical symptoms than those without grade 4 CIN. It was also noted that the negative impacts on quality of life lingered even after the ANC had improved [4–6].

5. Herbal treatments used among cancer patients suffering from neutropenia

In China, herbal remedies have been used for over two thousand years, making Chinese herbal medicine (CHM) an integral part of the country's healthcare system.

One of the major tenets of Chinese medicine is the concept of "treat pre-disease," or the prevention of disease before it manifests. Prevention of chemo-induced leukopenia and neutropenia may be greatly aided by CHM.

CHM has been found in recent research to reduce the negative side effects of conventional chemotherapy, while also providing personalised treatment programmes with multi-targeted and long-lasting effects. Furthermore, CHM has been shown to dramatically increase white blood cell counts in individuals with CIN in previous pharmacological investigations when used as an adjuvant treatment. Previous meta-analyses showed that when it comes to treating CIN caused by certain tumours, CHM is significantly more effective than traditional oral Western medication [1, 6, 7].

6. Neutropenia, infection, and antimicrobial stewardship

The overuse and misuse of antibiotics, as reported by the World Health Organisation, has resulted in the development of resistance, which threatens global health security. Mortality, medical care utilisation, and treatment-related expenses all rise when patients contract infections caused by multidrug-resistant (MDR) bacteria. Cancer patients often succumb to infections as their disease progresses. Moreover, as microbial resistance patterns shift, treating infections in people with neutropenia becomes more difficult [10, 11]. Because of the need to treat neutropenia over a lengthy period of time, doctors often prescribe many courses of broad-spectrum antibiotics, which puts strains of bacteria that are sensitive to the drugs under selection pressure and leads to an increase in multidrug-resistant strains. In patients with severe immunosuppression, bacterial translocation through intestinal mucosa is facilitated by compromised intestinal mucosal surfaces. This can lead to life-threatening infections [10, 11]. Therefore, it is essential matter to focus on the use of antimicrobial stewardship programmes among cancer patients suffering from neutropenia. The goals of Antimicrobial Stewardship programmes include lowering healthcare expenditures, improving the efficacy of treatment, and, most importantly, encouraging behaviours that lead to lower antibiotic resistance rates. Optimising antibiotic use is essential for lowering death and morbidity rates among these individuals. Formulary review, antibiotic restriction, audit, and feedback are all examples of broad antimicrobial treatments that have shown promise in patients with cancer [10, 11].

7. Cancer patients with neutropenic fever

Patients with an absolute neutrophil count of less than 500 cells per microliter, or an absolute neutrophil count that is expected to decrease to less than 500 cells per microliter within a 48-hour period, are considered to have febrile neutropenia if they experience either an oral temperature of greater than 38.3°C (approximately 100.9°F) at any given time, or a sustained temperature of greater than 38°C (100.4°F) for equal to or more than 1 hour [12, 13]. Neutropenia usually sets in around a week after cytotoxic treatment has been administered. Patients undergoing chemotherapy for solid tumours often experience neutropenia lasting fewer than 7 days, and only 5–30% experience febrile neutropenia, with the highest incidence happening during the first round of treatment [12, 13]. Patients undergoing precondition therapy for haematopoietic stem-cell transplantation or those undergoing chemotherapy for haematologic malignancies are more likely to experience more protracted neutropenia, lasting up to 14 days [12]. Therefore, more than 80% of patients taking chemotherapy for leukaemia or allogeneic haematopoietic stem-cell transplant will encounter at least one episode of febrile neutropenia. Only 40–50% of neutropenic fevers have an identifiable infectious aetiology, and only 10–30% of them have bacteraemia. However, empiric antibiotic coverage is necessary immediately for all patients presenting with febrile neutropenia [12, 13]. This is because there now exist no diagnostic tests or scoring systems that can accurately differentiate between people with bacteraemia and those without the infection. Accordingly, all patients must be provided the advantage of initial empiric therapy that predominantly covers the gram-negative infections that represent the greatest concern to them. Translocation of intestinal bacteria into the circulation is the most common cause of bacteraemia in this population [12, 13]. It has traditionally been difficult to distinguish bacteremias generated by catheters from those that began in the gut, despite the fact that catheter-related bloodstream infections constitute a prominent cause of infection in patients with febrile neutropenia [13, 14]. To better compare central line-associated bloodstream infection rates between cancer and noncancer centres, the National Healthcare Safety Network recently developed a new surveillance definition of mucosal barrier injury-associated laboratory-confirmed bloodstream infection to distinguish bloodstream infections caused by oral or intestinal microbiota in patients with cancer from those that are catheter related [13, 14]. These definitions apply to individuals with a bloodstream infection caused by a microorganism that is known to colonise the gastrointestinal system, who are neutropenic or who have undergone a transplant. In neutropenic cancer patients, gram-negative rods like Enterobacteriaceae (which includes *Escherichia coli*, *Klebsiella* species, and *Enterobacter* species) and *Pseudomonas aeruginosa* have traditionally been the most common pathogens causing bloodstream infections, but gram-positive organisms like *coagulase-negative staphylococci* and *viridans* group streptococci have recently become more common [12–14]. Empiric therapy for febrile neutropenia, however, should focus on gram-negative bacteria because of the high mortality and morbidity rates associated with gram-negative sepsis. Patients with neutropenia who do not get empiric antibiotics have a death rate of up to 70% when exposed to unopposed gram-negative bacteraemia [12–14]. Patients with neutropenic fever who are given empiric antibiotic therapies, on the other hand, have a mortality rate anywhere from 4% to 20%, depending on the severity of their underlying conditions and the presence or absence of gram-negative rod bacteraemia and/or tissue-invasive infections like pneumonia [12, 15, 16]. The underlying cancer and the cumulative treatment also alter the risk and range of infection. In general, the risk of infectious problems is higher for patients with refractory illness who have undergone numerous lines of chemotherapy and have experienced extended neutropenia. Infection can also be spread by tumours, particularly those in the intestine because they can block off passageways or enter already contaminated areas [12, 15, 16].

8. Preliminary assessment

Patients who exhibit febrile neutropenia should undergo the collection of a minimum of two sets of blood cultures. It is preferable for one set to be obtained through a peripheral venipuncture, and if available, the other set should be obtained from a central venous catheter [12, 17, 18]. Following this, the administration of empiric antibiotics should be initiated, with specific regimens to be discussed at a later point. It is recommended that the patient undergo a comprehensive assessment of their medical history and a thorough physical examination. There are several significant factors that should be taken into account when considering the patient's medical history [12, 17, 18]. These factors include conducting a thorough review of the patient's bodily systems, assessing any existing medical comorbidities, examining the specific chemotherapy regimen and the timing of the most recent chemotherapy cycle, evaluating any previous infections, considering recent antibiotic prophylaxis or therapy, identifying potential exposure to ill individuals, and examining the patient's social history [12, 17, 18]. The comprehensive assessment should encompass a thorough evaluation of various areas, such as the integumentary system, catheter insertion sites, respiratory system, sinuses, oral cavity, abdominal region, perirectal area, and neurologic system. These specific regions are of particular importance as they may serve as potential reservoirs for infectious agents in patients experiencing neutropenia as a result of chemotherapy [12, 17, 18]. It is recommended to conduct regular laboratory tests, such as complete blood count (CBC) with differential and comprehensive metabolic panel. Additionally, a symptom-oriented investigation should be pursued, involving cultures and/or imaging procedures. Patients presenting with respiratory symptoms should undergo a diagnostic evaluation that includes a chest radiograph or computed tomography scan, as well as a sputum culture if feasible. Additionally, it is advisable to consider respiratory viral testing, especially during the influenza season [12, 17, 18].

9. Analysis of risks

The publication of the Multinational Association for Supportive Care in Cancer (MASCC) risk index score in 2000 aimed to identify patients who, upon initial presentation with febrile neutropenia, exhibit a low risk for mortality and other severe complications throughout the subsequent duration of neutropenia [12, 17, 18]. By promptly identifying individuals who are at low or high risk for complications, it becomes feasible to formulate less intensive empiric antibiotic management protocols for the low-risk cohort, such as prescribing oral and/or outpatient antibiotics [12, 17, 18]. The components of the weighted MASCC scoring system consist of the following factors: the severity of symptoms associated with febrile neutropenia upon initial presentation, the presence of hypotension, a medical history of pulmonary disease, a history of fungal infection, dehydration, the patient's age, and whether the patient is receiving outpatient or inpatient care at the onset of febrile neutropenia [12, 17, 18].

10. The initial empirical therapy

Patients who have a high MASCC score, indicating a low-risk level, and are scheduled for outpatient treatment typically receive intravenous antibiotics following the collection of blood cultures. In such cases, it is possible to administer an oral treatment regimen consisting of ciprofloxacin combined with amoxicillin-clavulanic acid, levofloxacin, or moxifloxacin. In addition, patients have the option to receive intravenous antibiotic treatment in a home or outpatient setting [12, 15].

It is recommended that patients undergo daily evaluation within the initial 72-hour period. Additionally, patients should receive counselling regarding the necessity of returning if their blood cultures yield positive results, if they exhibit new signs or symptoms, or if they experience persistent or recurrent fever beyond a duration of 3 to 5 days [12, 15]. It is important to mention that individuals who are currently undergoing oral fluoroquinolone prophylaxis are not eligible for treatment with oral agents. Patients who are experiencing fever and neutropenia but do not satisfy the low-risk MASCC criteria, which require a score of less than 21 points, are classified as being at a heightened risk for complications during their subsequent period of neutropenia [12, 15]. While the MASCC scoring system does not consider the duration of neutropenia as a risk factor, our standard procedure is to admit all patients undergoing chemotherapy, particularly those with acute myelogenous leukaemia or undergoing stem-cell transplantation, which are anticipated to experience a period of low absolute neutrophil counts lasting longer than one week (less than 500 cell per microliter) [12, 15].

Patients who are at high risk should be admitted to the hospital in order to undergo thorough evaluation and receive appropriate treatment for potential infection. The duration of this procedure should not exceed one hour, encompassing the time from the initial presentation to the subsequent administration of antibiotics [12, 19]. It is crucial to minimise any delays in this process, as research has demonstrated a correlation between prolonged waiting times and unfavourable patient outcomes. It is recommended that patients be promptly administered a broad-spectrum parenteral antibiotic that possesses antipseudomonal activity [12, 19]. Two management strategies, namely escalation and de-escalation, have been delineated for the treatment of these patients. The de-escalation strategy involves an initial therapy regimen that incorporates treatment for multidrug-resistant gram-negative rods and gram-positive cocci [12, 19]. This may include the administration of a combination of carbapenem, aminoglycoside, and glycopeptide medications. This comprehensive therapeutic approach is commonly reserved for patients who exhibit severe sepsis or are identified as being colonised with bacteria that are resistant to treatment. Upon the patient's improvement and the absence of multi-drug-resistant organisms in the cultures, it is possible to de-escalate the treatment to a more targeted approach [12, 18, 19]. In the context of febrile neutropenia, stable patients are commonly managed using an escalation approach. This involves initiating treatment with b-lactam monotherapy, and subsequently incorporating additional agents if warranted by culture data or clinical deterioration [12]. The agents that are commonly recommended and have been demonstrated to be effective include cefepime, piperacillin-tazobactam, ceftazidime, or carbapenem with activity against pseudomonas (imipenem or meropenem). The selection of monotherapy should be influenced by prior infections and susceptibility patterns, along with the availability of institutional antibiograms [12, 18, 19]. When selecting therapy, it is crucial to take into account symptoms, complaints, and findings from physical examination. For instance, individuals experiencing abdominal symptoms, such as abdominal pain or diarrhoea, may require anaerobic protection. In such cases, it is recommended to administer piperacillin-tazobactam as the primary empirical therapy or to supplement cefepime with metronidazole [12, 18, 19]. Despite the fact that antipseudomonal carbapenems possess remarkable efficacy against anaerobic pathogens, their utilisation is most appropriate for the management of complex infections caused by drug-resistant microorganisms, specifically extended-spectrum β-lactamase-producing Enterobacteriaceae [12, 18, 19]. Based on the antibiogram profiles of various sites, which indicate the extent of carbapenem efficacy against gram-negative pathogens, the utilisation of carbapenems may be deemed appropriate for the treatment of sepsis in neutropenic patients. Routine coverage of uncomplicated, stable patients does not warrant the recommendation of carbapenems [12, 18, 19]. The implementation of fluoroquinolone prophylaxis has resulted in a decrease in the incidence of infections caused by gram-negative rods. Nevertheless, fluoroquinolones are frequently linked to higher rates of multidrug-resistant organisms, which consequently exposes patients to the possibility of breakthrough infections that may be less responsive to antibiotic therapy [12, 18, 19]. Furthermore, the majority of studies fail to exhibit a notable enhancement in overall survival when employing prophylaxis, thus leading to variations in prophylactic practises across different centres. In healthcare facilities where fluoroquinolone prophylaxis is implemented, it is crucial to maintain a high level of vigilance in order to detect and address the presence of multidrug-resistant organisms [12, 18, 19]. In the last three decades, there has been an increase in the prevalence of gram-positive bacteremias. However, it is noteworthy that these infections seldom lead to swift mortality in individuals experiencing febrile neutropenia, except in cases involving viridans group streptococci [12, 18, 19]. Hence, in the case of patients who are stable and do not exhibit sepsis, pneumonia, mucositis, or any indication of line infection, there is no advantage in the empirical inclusion of vancomycin to the initial regimen employed for the treatment of neutropenic fever. There are multiple clinical practise guidelines available to assist in the management of febrile neutropenia [12, 18, 19].

11. Conclusion

The rates of mortality and morbidity linked to neutropenia are significantly elevated. Hence, it is imperative that the administration of treatment be entrusted to a collective of medical professionals, including physicians, nurses, and chemists. It is advisable to seek recommendations for treatment alternatives, such as antibiotics and antifungals, from healthcare professionals specialising in infectious diseases, internal medicine, or paediatrics. Regular monitoring of a patient with severe neutropenia is imperative due to its potentially life-threatening nature. Key aspects to be assessed include the total blood cell count, blood chemistry, infectious disease indicators, and immunotherapy. During the period of awaiting the outcomes, it is imperative to initiate an empirical therapy, specifically the administration of an antibiotic. Subsequently, based on the outcomes of the assessment, the physician will determine whether to proceed with the empirical therapy that has been administered or to prescribe appropriate treatment(s).

12. Recommendations

It is highly imperative for future studies to focus on developing treatments that can be used to prevent the incidence of such a critical medical issue, specifically among cancer patients. Mainly to prevent the incidence of other major medical issues (which can delay the administration of chemotherapy or reduce the dose) and to maintain cancer patient's QOL within the required level.

Author details

Bassam Abdul Rasool Hassan[1*] and Ali Haider Mohammed[2]

1 Department of Pharmacy, Al Rafidain University College, Baghdad, Iraq

2 School of Pharmacy, Monash University Malaysia, Selangor, Malaysia

*Address all correspondence to: bassamsunny@yahoo.com

References

[1] Wang Q, Ye H, Wang Q, Li W, Yu B, Bai Y, et al. Chinese herbal medicine for chemotherapy-induced leukopenia: A systematic review and meta-analysis of high-quality randomized controlled trials. Frontiers in Pharmacology. 2021;**12**:1-15. DOI: 10.3389/fphar.2021.573500

[2] Carson-Dewitt R. Cancer. In: Longe JL, editor. The Gale Encyclopedia of Medicine. Farmington Hills: Gale Group; 2002

[3] Markman M. Principles of cancer screening. In: Aziz K, Wu GY, editors. Cancer Screening a Practical Guide for Physicians. New Jersey: Humana Press; 2002

[4] Angel A, Justiz Vaillant, Patrick M. Zito. Neutropenia [Internet]. 2023. Available from: https://www.ncbi.nlm.nih.gov/books/NBK507702/

[5] Geraldine P, PhD ME, Ropka. Quality of life and chemotherapy-induced neutropenia. Cancer Nursing. 2005;**3**:167-171. DOI: 10.1097/00002820-200505000-00001

[6] Dolan S. Leucopenia and neutropenia. In: Brighton D, Wood M, editors. The Royal Marsden Hospital Handbook of Cancer Chemotherapy. Churchill Livingstone: Elsevier; 2005

[7] Dale DC. Neutropenia. In: Herman NW, editor. Encyclopedia of Life's Sciences. Chichester: John Wiley & Son's, Ltd; 2005

[8] Sapkota B, Shrestha R, Chapagai S, Shakya DK, Bista P. Validation of risk of chemotherapy-induced neutropenia: Experience from oncology hospital of Nepal. Cancer Management and Research. 2020;**12**:3751-3758. DOI: 10.2147/CMAR.S243916

[9] Bledsoe BE, Kufs D, Soltis CA. Hematology. In: Bledsoe BE, Porter RS, Cherry RA, editors. Paramedic Care/ Principles and Practice. New Jersey: Pearson Prentice Hall; 2005

[10] Alves J, Abreu B, Palma P, Alp E, Vieceli T, Rello J. Antimicrobial stewardship on patients with neutropenia: A narrative review commissioned by microorganisms. Microorganisms. 2023;**11**:1-18. DOI: 10.3390/microorganisms11051127

[11] Keck JM, Wingler MJB, Cretella DA, Vijayvargiya P, Wagner JL, Barber KE, et al. Approach to fever in patients with neutropenia: A review of diagnosis and management. Therapeutic Advances in Infectious Disease. 2022;**9**:1-17. DOI: 10.1177/20499361221138346

[12] Andrea JZ, Alison GF. Optimal management of neutropenic fever in patients with cancer. Journal of Oncology Practice. 2019;**15**:19-24. DOI: 10.1200/JOP.18.00269

[13] Philip AP. Management of patients with fever and neutropenia through the arc of time. Annals of Internal Medicine. 2019;**170**(6):389-397. DOI: 10.7326/M18-3192

[14] Wijeratne DT, Wright K, Gyawali B. Risk-stratifying treatment strategies for febrile neutropenia—Tools, tools everywhere, and not a single one that works? JCO Oncology Practice. 2021;**17**(11):651-655. DOI: 10.1200/OP.21.00148

[15] Ishikawa K, Masaki T, Kawai F, Ota E, Mori N. Systematic review of the

short-term versus long-term duration of antibiotic Management for Neutropenic Fever in patients with Cancer. Cancers. 2023;**15**:1-15. DOI: 10.3390/cancers15051611

[16] Klastersky J, Paesmans M, Aoun M, Georgala A, Loizidou A, Lalami Y, et al. Clinical research in febrile neutropenia in cancer patients: Past achievements and perspectives for the future. World Journal of Clinical Infectious Diseases. 2016;**6**(3):37-60. DOI: 10.5495/wjcid.v6.i3.37

[17] Dale DC. How I diagnose and treat neutropenia. Current Opinion in Hematology. 2016;**23**(1):1-4. DOI: 10.1097/MOH.0000000000000208

[18] Boeriu E, Borda A, Vulcanescu DD, Sarbu V, Arghirescu ST, Ciorica O, et al. Diagnosis and Management of Febrile Neutropenia in pediatric oncology patients. A Systematic Review. Diagnostics. 2022;**12**:1-12. DOI: 10.3390/diagnostics12081800

[19] Anat S, Elena C, Roni B, Dafna Y, Leonard L, Mical P. Early discontinuation of antibiotics for febrile neutropenia versus continuation until neutropenia resolution in people with cancer. Cochrane Database of Systematic Reviews. 2019;**1**:1-49. DOI: 10.1002/14651858.CD012184.pub2

Chapter 5

Toll-Like Receptors as a New Era in Cancer Therapy

Mohammed AW. Almorish and Ali A. Alyahawi

Abstract

Toll-like receptors (TLRs) are crucial in immune response by detecting pathogen and host molecules, connecting innate and adaptive immunity. They trigger the expression of various proteins and kinases, leading to the production of inflammatory mediators. Research suggests TLRs are potential targets for treating inflammation-related diseases, autoimmune diseases, infections, and cancers, with TLR antagonists showing efficacy in pre-clinical and clinical settings. The modulation of immune responses by TLRs has led to their consideration as targets for cancer therapy, showing protective effects against different cancer types. This chapter discusses the potential of TLR-based therapies in cancer treatment, including both established and emerging discoveries.

Keywords: toll-like receptors, cancer therapy, imiquimod, TLR3, entolimod

1. Introduction

Cancer constitutes the leading cause of death among humans, representing one out of every six deaths worldwide [1]. The World Health Organization (WHO) indicates that approximately 10 million fatalities were linked to cancer in the year 2020, with the mortality rate exhibiting a persistent increase [1]. Advancements in diagnostic methodologies have enabled the detection of an array of cancer types. Nearly all anatomical regions are vulnerable to tumorigenesis, and the neoplastic growth across various organs is widely recognized as a critical contributor to the most fatal cancer types [1, 2]. As per the statistics available until 2020, colorectal and rectal cancer, prostate cancer, non-melanoma skin cancer, breast cancer, lung cancer, and gastric cancer collectively account for roughly 2.26, 2.21, 1.93, 1.41, 1.20, and 1.09% of the worldwide cancer incidence, respectively [3, 4]. In terms of mortality rates, lung cancer is documented as the most lethal form, followed by colorectal cancer, liver cancer, gastric cancer, and ductal carcinoma [3]. Furthermore, approximately four thousand pediatric cases are diagnosed with cancer each year, with cervical cancer identified as one of the most common types of malignancy [3].

1.1 TLR structures and ligands

TLR constitutes a type I transmembrane protein characterized by three principal structural domains. The protein features a Leucine-rich repeat (LRR) within its extracellular domain, a membrane-embedded structural domain, and a Toll/IL-1R (TIR) homology domain located in the cytoplasm [4].

Toll-like receptors (TLRs) function as receptors of the innate immune system that interact with pathogenic ligands, thereby initiating inflammatory cascades [4, 5]. In mammals, a total of 13 TLRs (TLR 1-13) have been recognized, which are classified into two groups: extracellular (TLR1, TLR2, TLR4, TLR5, TLR6, and TLR10) and intracellular (TLR3, TLR7, TLR8, and TLR9) [6, 7]. To date, ten functional TLRs have been documented in humans (TLR1–10), while 12 have been observed in murine models (TLR1–9 and TLR11–13). Each TLR consists of three distinct domains: extracellular LRR, transmembrane, and intracellular TIR [4, 5]. The extracellular domain of a TLR interacts with specific ligands via the co-receptor MD2 [8, 9].

Cell surface TLRs, including TLR1, TLR2, TLR4, TLR5, TLR6, and TLR10, primarily detect microbial membrane components. TLR2 forms dimers with other TLRs, enhancing the recognition of various PAMPs from diverse pathogens [9, 10]. Additionally, TLR2 identifies damage-associated molecular patterns (DAMPs) produced by necrosis and inflammation. Dendritic cells and macrophages release pro-inflammatory cytokines upon TLR ligand activation. TLR4 recognizes lipopolysaccharides and MD2, forming a TLR4–MD2–LPS dimer. LPS, prevalent in Gram-negative bacteria, is a potent immunostimulant linked to septic shock. TLR4 also detects other pathogenic factors, activating inflammatory cytokine production and IFN responses. For example, TLR4 identifies viral capsid proteins and virulent proteins from *Streptococcus pneumoniae*. TLR5 recognizes flagellin, particularly in the small intestine's DCs, triggering inflammatory mediators and immune responses (**Figure 1**) [9–13].

Within the intracellular organelles such as lysosomes, endosomes, and the endoplasmic reticulum exhibit the presence of TLRs, including TLR3, TLR7, TLR8, and TLR9, which are instrumental in the recognition of nucleic acids derived from pathogens and in the context of autoimmunity. These TLRs stimulate IFN and cytokine production, initiating antiviral responses. TLR3 detects RNA from damaged cells and viral dsRNA, activating NF-κB and ensuing IFN and pro-inflammatory cytokine production. TLR7, found in pDCs, recognizes viral ssRNA and bacterial RNA, promoting type I IFN and pro-inflammatory cytokines. Human TLR8 responds to viral and bacterial RNA, showing similarity to TLR7, with heightened expression in monocytes after stimulation. TLR9 identifies bacterial and viral DNA rich in unmethylated CpG motifs, crucial for IFN-α production in pDCs during DNA virus infections like HSV-1 and HSV-2 [11, 13].

The functions and ligand recognition of human TLRs 1–9 are well understood. In contrast, TLR10 is poorly characterized due to the lack of suitable murine models, as retroviral insertion does not result in functional TLR10 expression. While TLRs generally promote pro-inflammatory cytokines, TLR10 has been shown to elicit anti-inflammatory responses. Its anti-inflammatory mechanism may involve competition with other TLRs for ligands or the promotion of anti-inflammatory cytokines [11, 13].

TLRs 11, 12, and 13 are present in mice but not in humans, and their functions are not well defined. TLR11 is found in the endolysosome and can detect protein structures from *Toxoplasma gondii* and components of uropathogenic *E. coli*. Similarly, TLR12 is located in bone marrow cells and can recognize proteins from *T. gondii*. TLR13 identifies bacterial 23S rRNA and regulates the innate immune response [11, 13].

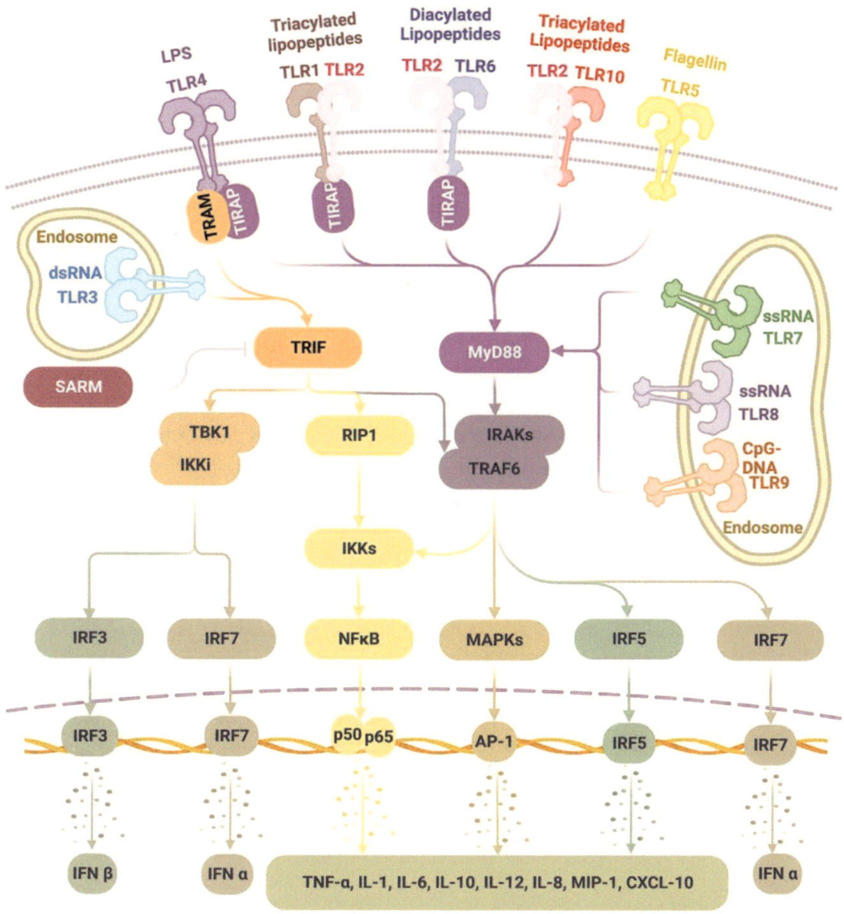

Figure 1.
TLR ligands and signaling pathways: In a physiological context, TLRs are located on the cell membrane (specifically TLRs 1, 2, 4, 5, 6, and 10) or within the endosomal compartment (namely TLRs 3, 7, 8, and 9). These receptors are capable of identifying a diverse array of pathogen-associated molecular patterns (PAMPs). Following ligand binding, dimerization of TLRs can trigger the activation of either the MyD88 or TRIF signaling pathways. Notably, TLR4 can engage both MyD88 (utilizing the adaptor protein TIRAP) and TRIF (with the adaptor protein TRAM) pathways; TLR3 exclusively activates TRIF, while TLRs 1/2, 2/6, 2/10, 5, and TLRs 79 engage MyD88 independently, all without the necessity of an adaptor protein. Consequently, type I interferons (IFNs) are produced through the activation of IRF3 and IRF7, alongside the production of inflammatory cytokines mediated by NF-kB, MAPKs, and IRF5, thereby initiating a broad spectrum of inflammatory and immune responses, which underpins the potential for therapeutic investigation of TLRs in cancer treatment [11].

1.2 TLR- pathways

The interaction of ligands triggers structural modifications within the TIR domain, thereby enhancing the recruitment of adaptor proteins such as MyD88 and TRIF. TIRAP facilitates the association of MyD88 with TLR2 and TLR4, leading to the activation of NF-kB and MAPKs [6, 8]. Conversely, TRIF binding to TLR3/4 induces IRF-3, NF-kB, and MAPK proliferation [8, 9]. LPS binding to TLR4-MD2 can trigger MyD88-dependent or independent signaling cascades [6, 10]. With the exception of TLR3, TLRs primarily utilize MyD88 for downstream signaling, which is prevalent in immune and cancer cells [12, 13]. Research indicates that MyD88 and its pathways significantly influence cancer progression, prompting its expression as a prognostic marker for various human cancers (**Figure 1**) [14–16].

1.3 The involvement of TLRs in cancer

Toll-like receptors (TLRs) exhibit significant overexpression in various malignancies, with specific TLRs associated with distinct cancer types, while their expression correlates negatively with clinical findings in head and neck squamous cell carcinoma [17]. Moreover, the aberrant localization of TLRs, such as TLR2, TLR4, and TLR5 in colorectal cancer cells, further underscores the complexities of their role in tumor biology [18].

TLRs exhibit bifunctional characteristics in the context of neoplasia, influencing the dynamics of tumor advancement and inhibition in a manner that is contingent upon the specific receptor subtype. For example, TLR4 is known to enhance antitumor immunity in hepatoblastoma, yet conversely facilitates tumor proliferation in hepatocellular carcinoma and cervical carcinoma [19]. The antitumor pathways activated by TLRs encompass the secretion of pro-inflammatory cytokines and the induction of apoptosis in tumor cells, whereas their pro-tumor activities enhance cellular proliferation, survival, and metastasis and contribute to an immunosuppressive environment [16]. Moreover, TLRs are implicated in the activation of regulatory T cells, which cultivate an immune environment conducive to tumor survival. The contrasting influences exerted by TLRs arise from variations in receptor expression and responsiveness within tumor cells and their surrounding microenvironment [17, 20]. Consequently, it is essential to approach TLRs and tumor entities with a nuanced perspective; ascertaining the particular effects of each TLR in therapeutic frameworks is imperative, since certain patients may derive greater benefits from TLR antagonists while others might respond more favorably to agonists.

1.4 Targeting of TLRs in cancer therapy

Preclinical and initial clinical investigations into TLR therapies for solid tumors have demonstrated notable antitumor efficacy. The TLR7/8 agonist MBS8 elicited the production of cytokine IP-10 while exhibiting minimal TNF-α and IFN-γ levels, showcasing its monotherapeutic potential and ability to overcome anti-PD-1 resistance in murine models. Comparable antitumor effects were observed with TLR7 agonists, such as resiquimod and guretolimod (DSP-0509) [21–23].

To date, regulatory bodies have yet to approve a TLR antagonist for cancer treatment. However, the FDA has sanctioned two vaccines featuring TLR agonist adjuvants: monophosphoryl lipid A (MPLA) and bacillus Calmette-Guérin (BCG) [24, 25]. MPLA, a TLR4 ligand isolated from *Salmonella minnesota*, augments immune responses against human papillomavirus strains 16 and 18, whereas BCG, an agonist of TLR2/4, is employed as an intravesical immunotherapeutic agent for non-muscle-invasive bladder carcinoma [26]. Furthermore, imiquimod, functioning as a TLR7 agonist, is applied topically for the treatment of superficial basal cell carcinoma, thereby enhancing antitumor immunity via the activation of macrophages and dendritic cells [24, 25].

TLR agonists may transform "cold tumors" into "hot tumors" with enhanced immunological responses, leading to improved patient outcomes with immune checkpoint inhibitors, thus prompting an investigation into their application as independent therapeutic modalities, in conjunction with other treatment regimens and as adjuvant components in vaccines for a range of solid neoplasms (**Figure 2**).

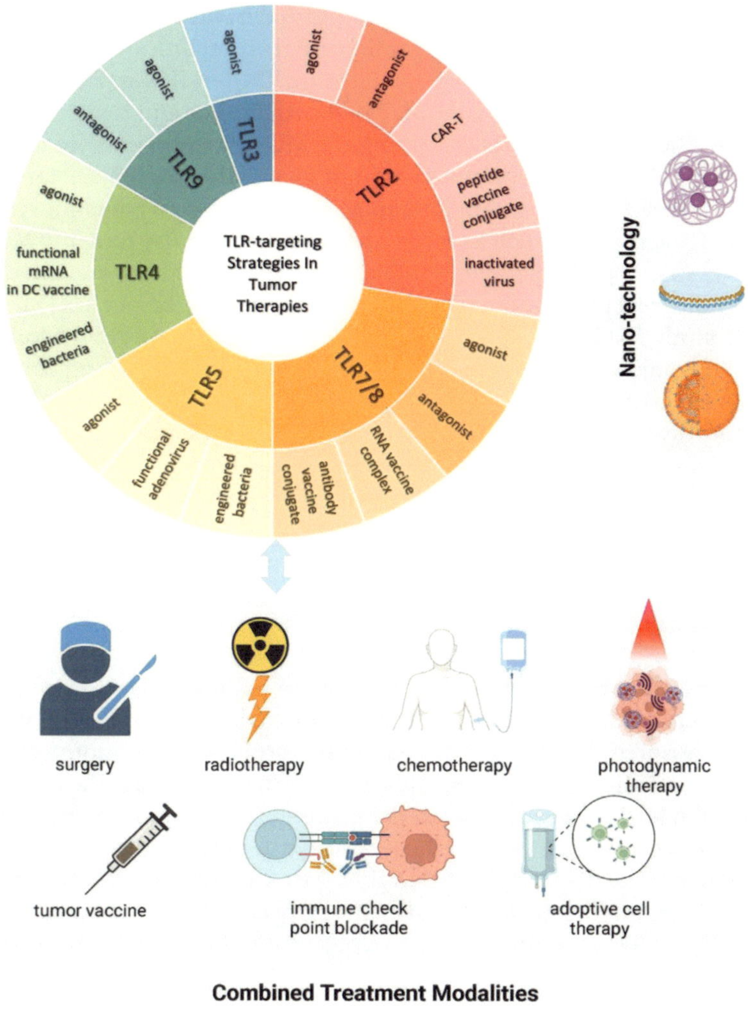

Figure 2.
Strategies targeting TLR and their integration in cancer treatment modalities. Current tumor therapy strategies targeting TLRs involve the creation of novel TLR agonists, inactivated viruses, engineered bacteria, functional RNAs, vaccine conjugates, modified T cells, and TLR antagonism, with a growing integration of nanotechnology for enhanced drug efficacy and safety, while emerging evidence highlights the necessity for multi-agent and multi-modality approaches to overcome tumor-induced immunosuppression.

1.5 TLR agonists in clinical development

1.5.1 TLR2/TLR4 agonists

Bacillus Calmette-Guerin (BCG) is a pioneering TLR agonist for oncological therapies. BCG received FDA approval over four decades ago for bladder cancer treatment. Its anti-cancer mechanism involves dual TLR2 and TLR4 activation. BCG's role as an adjuvant has been extensively evaluated in melanoma and colorectal cancer [27, 28]. A Phase III trial of Canvaxin, a melanoma vaccine with BCG, did not enhance survival outcomes despite initial promise. Conversely, BCG monotherapy showed improved efficacy in patients with advanced melanoma in the same trial. OncoVAX, an autologous colon cancer vaccine with BCG, demonstrated significant survival benefits in a

Phase II study [29, 30]. Similarly, OM-174, a lipid A derivative, is under investigation as a vaccine adjuvant for melanoma and solid tumors. Preclinical studies suggest that OM-174's therapeutic activity is linked to increased TNF-a, IFN-g, and iNOS [31, 32]. Monophosphoryl lipid A (MPL), another TLR4 activator, is employed in various vaccines as an adjuvant. Stimuvax, targeting the MUC1 tumor antigen, uses MPL but failed to show significant therapeutic benefit in Phase III trials [33]. A cancer vaccine targeting the MAGE A3 antigen employs an MPL-based mixed adjuvant system [34]. Additional TLR4 activators, such as AS04 and GLA-SE, are also under investigation in clinical studies [35, 36]. Meanwhile, lipoteichoic acids from Gram-negative bacteria can activate TLR2 receptors and induce anti-tumor immune responses [21, 24].

A Phase 1 study (NCT03447314) evaluating the intravenous TLR4 agonist GSK1795091 in conjunction with various immunotherapies, including pembrolizumab, has been completed, though biological activity variations arose due to manufacturing modifications [37]. Out of 54 patients treated, a significant majority (94%) reported at least one Grade 1/2 treatment-emergent adverse event (TEAE), with notable occurrences of chills, nausea, and fatigue. Despite limited data, three patients exhibited a partial response, while 13 achieved stable disease, alongside observed pharmacodynamic responses for certain cytokines, excluding TNF-α [37].

1.5.2 TLR5 agonists

TLR5 is stimulated by flagellin, with its derivatives being investigated for their anticancer effects. CBLB502, which is derived from Salmonella flagellin, is currently undergoing assessment for its efficacy against squamous cell carcinoma of the head and neck in phase I clinical trials [38]. Research has indicated that the activation of TLR5 by flagellin leads to a reduction in the proliferation of immunogenic tumors, while having no significant effect on those with weak immunogenicity. These findings arise from the disparity between IFN-g:IL-4 ratios and the population of CD4 + CD25+ T regulatory cells. Moreover, an early combination treatment involving flagellin and CpG ODNs resulted in the complete inhibition of tumor growth [39].

1.5.2.1 Mobilan

Mobilan (M-VM3), a recombinant adenovirus encoding flagellin, has been studied for prostate cancer treatment. To enhance TLR5 agonism in TLR5-negative tumors, the adenoviral construct Mobilan (M-VM3), encoding the TLR5 receptor and its agonist, was engineered, demonstrating notable preclinical efficacy in prostate cancer models, while its safety profile was validated in phase I trial (NCT02654938) with results pending [40]. Flagellin treatment in breast cancer cells has been shown to inhibit cell proliferation and tumor growth [41].

1.5.2.2 Entolimod

Entolimod (CBLB502), a TLR5 agonist derived from Salmonella flagellin, was administered via subcutaneous injection in a phase 1 clinical trial involving 26 participants with advanced cancers. Reported adverse effects included temporary hypotension, elevated blood glucose levels, and fever, with few instances of severe adverse reactions documented. Entolimod elicited the release of IL-6, IL-8, and IL-10 while diminishing the population of immunosuppressive cells; however, no tumor responses were observed [42]. A randomized phase 2 clinical trial assessing entolimod for colorectal cancer was launched in Russia, but its present status remains uncertain [43]. Mett et al. have engineered GP532, a modified TLR5 agonist designed to attenuate neutralizing antibody responses while preserving pro-inflammatory activities, although its anti-tumor effectiveness has yet to be evaluated in clinical trials [44].

A recent study demonstrates that the syngeneic 4 T1 mammary carcinoma model for refractory triple-negative breast cancer exhibited improved survival rates when treated intra-tumorally with TLR5 agonists combined with CTLA-4 and PD-1 targeting antibodies. Additionally, long-term survivors displayed immunologic memory upon tumor re-challenge, with distinct cytokine profiles and potential biomarkers indicating enhanced survival, suggesting that this combination therapy may be an effective strategy for ICT-refractory solid tumors [45]. Presently, no active clinical trials involving entolimod as an anticancer agent exist.

1.5.3 TLR3 agonists

The identification of TLR3 activation by means of double-stranded RNA was initially reported by Alexopoulou et al. [46]. At present, polyinosinic-polycytidylic acid (poly(I:C)) serves as a TLR3 agonist, markedly augmenting dendritic cell activation, which in turn enhances antigen presentation for CD8+ cytotoxic T cells. Furthermore, it promotes the indirect activation of natural killer cells and T cells, thereby inducing robust anti-tumor immune responses [47, 48].

Consequently, poly(I:C) is commonly employed in cancer vaccine formulations; however, due to its rapid degradation and toxicological concerns, several stable derivatives, such as Hiltonol (poly-ICLC), have been developed and evaluated in clinical trials for various solid tumors, which, while lacking significant anti-tumor efficacy, demonstrated satisfactory physiological safety [49, 50]. Despite limited anti-tumor efficacy in clinical trials, physiological safety was confirmed, while rintatolimod (Ampligen) has been approved for pancreatic cancer, triple-negative breast cancer, and brain tumors in conjunction with specific vaccines, and poly(I:C), and its derivatives are being explored as vaccine adjuvants for enhancing dendritic cell maturation and Th1 cytokine expression in ongoing clinical investigations [51, 52].

1.5.3.1 Ampligen

NCT03734692 (phase I/II) examines the effectiveness of a chemoimmunotherapy regimen that integrates intensive locoregional intraperitoneal cisplatin, intraperitoneal ampligen, and intravenous pembrolizumab for individuals suffering from recurrent, platinum-sensitive ovarian carcinoma. Participants are subjected to six treatment cycles at three-week intervals, succeeded by laparoscopic cytoreduction approximately four weeks subsequent to the fourth cycle, with further treatments administered in the postoperative period [53]. Preliminary results from Radolec et al. indicate that among 17 enrolled patients, the regimen was well tolerated, primarily inducing Grade 1 and 2 toxicities, and several patients exhibited remission with extended progression-free survival. In contrast, NCT04081389 (phase I) evaluates cytokine modulation therapy alongside standard chemotherapy in early-stage triple-negative breast cancer, employing celecoxib, intravenous recombinant IFN-α-2b, and intravenous ampligen over a structured timeline. Although this trial was temporarily halted for data analysis, results showed that the treatment was generally well tolerated, with mild adverse events and no dose-limiting toxicities. Notably, 56% of patients attained a pathologic complete response, with increased CD8α expression in tumor biopsies post-treatment, while other adverse events were observed that were not related to the study regimen [53–55].

1.5.3.2 Poly-ICLC

The NCT04116320 (phase I) study assesses the safety of focused ultrasound ablation with and without PD-1 blockade in conjunction with poly-ICLC for advanced solid tumors [56], while NCT04364230 (phase I/II) investigates the safety of a peptide vaccine combining six melanoma helper peptides and a mutated neoantigen peptide with local adjuvants such as CD40 antibody and poly-ICLC in melanoma patients, administered subcutaneously or intradermally at specified intervals [57].

1.5.3.3 BO-112

BO-112, a composite formulation of poly-IC in conjunction with polyethylenimine, is currently being examined in phase 2 clinical trial NCT04570332 to assess its safety and therapeutic efficacy in patients with advanced or metastatic melanoma who have exhibited disease progression following PD-1 blockade therapy [57]. The study involves administering pembrolizumab intravenously thrice weekly prior to BO-112, which is injected intratumorally for the initial seven weeks and subsequently every three weeks, with adjustments based on lesion detectability. Recruitment was concluded by August 14, 2021, involving 42 patients with confirmed disease progression, predominantly with cutaneous melanoma, and achieving an objective response rate of 27%. Safety assessments indicated a high incidence of treatment-related adverse events, with a significant proportion experiencing severe effects [58, 59].

1.5.3.4 Nexavant

Nexavant has emerged as a promising alternative to the TLR3 agonist poly(I:C) and its derivatives, showcasing unique physicochemical attributes and signaling mechanisms. It specifically activates TLR3 and RIG-I while circumventing MDA5, leading to pronounced immune responses and suppression of tumor growth in a variety of animal models, surpassing the efficacy of anti-PD-1 antibody therapies. The potential of Nexavant as a solitary anti-cancer agent or as part of combination therapies is particularly emphasized, especially regarding its effectiveness in augmenting immune cell recruitment and enhancing survival rates in metastatic scenarios [52].

1.5.4 TLR7 agonists

TLR7 functions as an endosomal sensor of the innate immune system, facilitating the synthesis of type I interferons (IFN-I) in addition to various pro-inflammatory cytokines upon detection of single-stranded RNA [60].

1.5.4.1 Imiquimod

Imiquimod (Aldara) has been approved by the FDA as a topical agent targeting TLR7 for superficial basal cell carcinoma (SCC) [61], with NCT04883645 evaluating its local and systemic safety, tolerability, and efficacy in early-stage oral SCC through self-administration in neoadjuvant settings, using quantitative multiplex immunofluorescence to analyze tumor samples for immunomodulatory effects [62].

1.5.4.2 TQ-A3334

TLR7 is known to detect viral ssRNA, and TQ-A3334, an oral TLR7 agonist, promotes the release of pro-inflammatory cytokines such as IFN-α and IP-10 [63]. A phase 1/2 trial (NCT04273815) investigating TQ-A3334 for non-small-cell lung cancer has shown that the drug is tolerable among healthy volunteers, with adverse events predominantly being minor and self-resolving [63]. Notably, cytokine levels returned to baseline within 72 hours post-treatment, underscoring the transient nature of the drug's immunomodulatory effects. The combination of TQ-A3334 and anti-PD-L1 therapy enhances tumor control and elevates CD8+ TIL frequency, indicating that TQ-A3334 effectively mobilizes innate immunity and boosts T cell infiltration in the tumor microenvironment, thereby augmenting the efficacy of anti-PD-L1 treatment in immune-deficient lung cancer [64].

1.5.4.3 LHC165

LHC165, an intratumoral TLR-7 agonist (NCT03301896) as a monotherapy and in conjunction with the PD-1 inhibitor spartalizumab, revealed treatment-emergent adverse events in 56% of participants, with notable incidences of pyrexia, injection site reactions, and other events across both treatment arms. The study was recently terminated by the Sponsor, with limited efficacy demonstrated by a partial response in 10% of the monotherapy cohort and 5% in the combination group. The study, which reported various grades of AEs and limited overall responses, was recently terminated by the Sponsor in August 2022 [65].

A recent study, a first-in-human phase I/Ib open-label, dose-escalation/expansion study, evaluated the safety, tolerability, pharmacokinetics, pharmacodynamics, and anti-tumor efficacy of LHC165 administered biweekly via intratumoral injection and in combination with spartalizumab in adults with advanced solid tumors, revealing acceptable safety profiles and limited anti-tumor activity [66].

1.5.4.4 BNT411

Intravenous BNT411 (NCT04101357) is currently being evaluated as a monotherapy for solid tumors and in combination with atezolizumab, carboplatin, and etoposide for patients with chemotherapy-naïve extensive-stage small-cell lung cancer. Among the cohort of 11 individuals administered monotherapy, there were reports of Grade 1/2 adverse events, alongside a singular case of Grade 3 pyrexia; however, no notable toxicities or severe adverse events were documented, and initial efficacy assessments suggested that one patient maintained stable disease for a duration of five months [67].

1.5.4.5 NJH395

Intravenous NJH395, an immune-enhancing antibody conjugate combines an uncharacterized TLR7 agonist with a monoclonal antibody that specifically targets the human epidermal growth factor receptor-2 (HER2). A phase 1 dose-escalation study demonstrated notable, though manageable, adverse effects, with 50% of participants displaying stable disease three weeks following infusion, in conjunction with an increase in tumor-infiltrating cytotoxic T lymphocytes [68].

Intravenous NJH395 represents an immune-enhancing antibody conjugate that combines a TLR7 agonist with a monoclonal antibody directed against the human epidermal growth factor receptor-2 (HER2). A phase 1 trial indicated that while significant adverse effects were observed, they were deemed manageable, and the treatment also enhanced tumor-infiltrating cytotoxic T cells, achieving stable disease in 50% of patients at three weeks [68]. Another study found results from 18 patients indicate effective TLR7 agonist delivery and IFN-I response modulation despite manageable cytokine release syndrome and notable challenges from antidrug antibodies and neuroinflammation at elevated doses [68, 69].

1.5.4.6 SHR2150

Ongoing first-in-human trials of TLR7 agonists include oral SHR2150 (NCT04588324) combined with chemotherapy and anti-PD-1 or anti-CD47 for advanced solid tumors, oral RO7119929 (NCT04338685) as a monotherapy for advanced hepatocellular carcinoma and liver metastases, and intravenous DSP-0509 (NCT03416335) both solo and with pembrolizumab for advanced solid tumors, with preliminary clinical data reported for some other TLR7 agonists [62, 70].

1.5.5 TLR7/8 agonists

1.5.5.1 BDB001

The Phase II trial NCT04819373 investigates the safety and efficacy of intravenous BDB001, created by Seven and Eight Biopharmaceuticals Inc., as a monotherapy for patients with anti-PD-1 or -PD-L1 refractory advanced solid tumors. Concurrently, phase I trial NCT04196530 evaluates the combination of intravenous BDB001 and atezolizumab in advanced solid tumor patients, revealing favorable tolerability and notable clinical responses among participants [71, 72]. Additionally, Phase II trial NCT03915678 examines the integration of BDB001 with atezolizumab and radiotherapy, with a structured treatment regimen emphasizing precise timing of administration and high-dose irradiation protocols [70].

1.5.5.2 BDB018

BDB018, an analog of BDB001, aims to amplify immune activation against cancer while ensuring a favorable safety profile, as evaluated in the phase I trial NCT04840394, which investigates the efficacy of intravenous BDB018 both as monotherapy and in combination with pembrolizumab in patients with unresectable or metastatic solid tumors that are either relapsed, refractory to standard care, or lack an approved treatment, encompassing a dose-escalation and expansion phase for the combination therapy [70–72].

1.5.5.3 BDC-1001

BDC-1001, like to the TLR7 agonist NJH395, functions as an immune-enhancing antibody conjugate integrating a HER2 monoclonal antibody that activates both TLR7 and TLR8. A phase 1/2 clinical trial (NCT04278144) is currently assessing BDC-1001's efficacy as a standalone treatment and in conjunction with pembrolizumab for HER2-positive advanced solid tumors, revealing a promising safety profile with manageable adverse events. Interim results indicate that, among 57 patients, the treatment was well tolerated, with notable cases of partial response and stable disease in various malignancies, suggesting potential therapeutic benefit [73, 74].

1.5.5.4 CV8102

CV8102, a type of non-coding RNA, augments innate immune responses via the TLR7/8 and retinoic acid-inducible gene I signaling pathways and is presently being evaluated both as a standalone treatment and in conjunction with a PD-1 antibody in a phase 1 clinical trial (NCT03291002) aimed at various advanced malignancies. Interim results indicated common adverse events including fatigue and fever, with notable efficacy observed in melanoma patients, showcasing both complete and partial responses, alongside varying outcomes in combination therapy [75]. Immunotherapy for hepatocellular carcinoma (HCC) shows considerable promise for improving clinical outcomes. The HepaVac-101 trial, a pioneering phase I/II multicenter study (NCT03203005), evaluates a combination of multipeptide antigens (IMA970A) and the TLR7/8/RIG I agonist CV8102, demonstrating a favorable safety profile and significant immune responses in a subset of patients, warranting further research into its therapeutic efficacy for HCC [76].

1.5.5.5 TransCon

Intratumoral TransCon TLR7/8 Agonist serves as a prodrug for the more efficacious resiquimod, which is a derivative of imiquimod. The design of TransCon TLR7/8 Agonist was specifically intended to facilitate localized retention, thereby reducing systemic side effects [77]. Presently, it is being assessed both as a standalone treatment and in conjunction with pembrolizumab in a phase 1/2 clinical trial (NCT04799054) that includes patients with advanced solid tumors. An interim analysis involving eight participants indicated the absence of dose-limiting toxicities or notable treatment-related systemic adverse events [77, 78]. The sole treatment-related adverse event documented was mild and transient reactions at the injection site.

1.5.6 TLR8 agonists

1.5.6.1 SBT6050

SBT6050 is a monoclonal antibody targeting HER2, linked to a TLR8 agonist, currently undergoing evaluation in various clinical trials. The study NCT05091528 has been terminated due to a strategic shift by the sponsor, while NCT04460456 aims to investigate the safety and efficacy of SBT6050, both as monotherapy and in conjunction with PD-1 inhibitors, in patients with HER2-positive malignancies. Initial outcomes from the latter trial indicate pharmacological activity across multiple dose levels, with observed adverse effects manageable through supportive intervention [79, 80].

1.5.6.2 SBT6290

SBT6290 comprises a monoclonal antibody against the tumor-associated antigen nectin-4, conjugated to a TLR8 agonist, which targets the overexpression of this adhesion molecule in various cancers and is currently being evaluated in the

NCT05234606 trial as a standalone treatment and in conjunction with pembrolizumab for Nectin-4 positive advanced solid tumors [81].

1.5.7 TLR9 agonist

TLR9 identifies unmethylated DNA sequences abundant in phosphate-linked CpG dinucleotides, which are prevalent in bacterial and viral genomes but scarce in mammals due to genomic methylation. Oligonucleotides are categorized into three classes: Class A enhances IFN-alpha production by plasmacytoid dendritic cells with limited B cell activation, while Class B has opposing effects, and Class C activates both cell types, combining features of Classes A and B [82, 83].

1.5.7.1 Lefitolimod

Lefitolimod (MGN1703), a TLR9 agonist, is currently under investigation in a phase 1 trial alongside ipilimumab for patients with advanced solid tumors due to unsatisfactory outcomes in the phase 3 IMPALA study. The IMPALA findings indicated comparable overall survival rates between lefitolimod and standard care, while safety assessments revealed no new adverse signals, with flu-like symptoms and injection site reactions being the most commonly reported treatment-related adverse events [84, 85].

1.5.7.2 Vidutolimod/CMP-001

Vidutolimod/CMP-001, a TLR9 agonist encapsulated within a virus-like particle, facilitates the expression of IFN-alpha in plasmacytoid dendritic cells and augments the production of IFN-inducible genes in T cells and NK cells [86]. Ongoing research is investigating its effectiveness as a standalone treatment and in combination with pembrolizumab for patients exhibiting resistance to PD-(L)1 inhibitors in a phase 1b clinical trial, which has demonstrated an overall response rate of 23% when used alongside pembrolizumab. The treatment's adverse effects were predominantly flu-like symptoms and hypotension, yet no treatment-related fatalities were reported [86, 87]. In a recently concluded phase 2 trial (NCT03618641), neoadjuvant therapy combining CMP-001 with nivolumab demonstrated a 70% pathologic response rate among 30 patients with stage IIIB-D melanoma, with significant correlations observed between biomarker profiles and intratumoral immune cell infiltration, despite some patients experiencing severe infusion-related adverse events leading to treatment discontinuation [88]. Ongoing and forthcoming studies are assessing CMP-001 in combination with various immune checkpoint inhibitors across a range of malignancies, which includes melanoma, recurrent/metastatic squamous cell carcinoma of the head and neck (SCCHN), metastatic colorectal cancer (CRC), pancreatic carcinoma, advanced nonmelanoma solid tumors, castration-resistant prostate cancer, and Merkel cell carcinoma. Additionally, a subcutaneous formulation is being explored; however, a trial evaluating the subcutaneous route alongside atezolizumab in patients with non-small-cell lung cancer (NSCLC) was discontinued due to insufficient therapeutic response [89].

1.5.7.3 SD-101

The Sponsor halted the development of SD-101, a Class C oligonucleotide, in 2019 due to a strategic restructuring, despite its promising anti-tumor efficacy in the

SYNERGY-001/KEYNOTE-184 trial with pembrolizumab [90]. Notably, the study revealed an overall response rate of 76% in metastatic melanoma patients receiving 2 mg of SD-101, alongside a notable T cell influx, while common adverse effects included injection site reactions and flu-like symptoms [91]. Responses were observed in both injected and non-injected lesions, as well as in tumors that were either PD-L1 positive or negative; among patients with recurrent or metastatic SCCHN, an overall response rate of 22% was noted for those receiving 2 mg of SD-101 and 26% for those receiving 8 mg, with treatment leading to a T cell influx in both tumor types and the most prevalent adverse events related to SD-101 being injection site reactions and flu-like symptoms [91, 92].

The ongoing clinical trials of SD-101 investigate its efficacy in various combinations, including nivolumab and radiation for chemotherapy-resistant metastatic pancreatic cancer (NCT04050085), pembrolizumab with androgen deprivation and stereotactic body radiation for newly diagnosed, hormone-naive oligometastatic prostate cancer (NCT03007732), nivolumab and ipilimumab for uveal melanoma (NCT04935229), neoadjuvant therapy with pembrolizumab for breast cancer (NCT01042379; I-SPY), pembrolizumab or nivolumab with ipilimumab for liver tumors (NCT05220722) and BMS986178 for solid tumors (NCT03831295) [70].

1.5.7.4 Cavrotolimod (AST-008)

Cavrotolimod (AST-008), a synthetic oligonucleotide, has been assessed in a terminated phase 1b/2 study (NCT03684785) for advanced solid tumors, where the phase 1b segment concluded enrollment revealing an overall objective response rate of 21% (4/19), including responses in two patients with Merkel cell carcinoma and two with melanoma, despite the study's administrative cessation [93]. Three of the four participants had prior disease progression on anti-PD-(L)1 therapy before entering the study; similar to tilsotolimod and CMP-001, cavrotolimod prompted regression of both injected and non-injected tumors with reactions at the injection site and symptoms resembling influenza being the predominant adverse effects, while its pharmacodynamic profile exhibited dose-dependent elevations in multiple cytokines (for instance, IP-10) and T cell infiltration in both treated and untreated lesions, whether administered independently or in combination with pembrolizumab [94].

1.5.7.5 Tilsotolimod (IMO-2125)

The intratumoral TLR9 agonist tilsotolimod (IMO-2125) effectively induces rapid elevations in IFN-γ and genes responsive to IFN following administration, exhibiting notable efficacy when administered in conjunction with ipilimumab in the ILLUMINATE-204 study. In this study, among 49 evaluable participants receiving the recommended phase 2 dosage (8 mg), the overall response rate was 22%, which included two complete responses and regression observed in both injected and non-injected lesions [95]. The combination regimen was generally manageable, with no adverse events resulting in discontinuation or mortality; however, nearly 48% of subjects reported severe adverse events, predominantly characterized by elevated liver enzymes and colitis. In the phase 1b ILLUMINATE-101 trial involving patients with solid tumors, the most frequently reported treatment-related adverse effects of tilsotolimod were fever, nausea, fatigue, chills, and vomiting. Conversely, the phase 3 ILLUMINATE-301 trial, which evaluated tilsotolimod alongside ipilimumab in patients with PD-1 inhibitor-refractory advanced melanoma, was halted due to lack of effectiveness, while ongoing investigations into the use of tilsotolimod in combined therapies for various solid tumors as well as its application as monotherapy in melanoma continue [83].

1.5.7.6 TAC-001

TAC-001 has received FDA approval as an investigational drug for the systemic treatment of advanced solid tumors. The ongoing phase I/II trial (NCT05399654, INCLINE-101) is designed to assess the safety, pharmacokinetics, and preliminary anti-tumor efficacy of TAC-001 administered intravenously in patients with advanced, metastatic, or recurrent solid tumors who have failed standard therapies [62].

2. Conclusions

The exploration of TLR agonists for cancer treatment is gaining traction among clinicians due to their potential to enhance anti-tumor immunity, as evidenced by ongoing clinical studies. Preliminary findings indicate that TLR7 and TLR9 agonists exhibit anti-tumor efficacy, both as monotherapies and in conjunction with established immune checkpoint inhibitors, particularly in resistant or PD-L1 negative cases. Importantly, while TLR agonists can elicit common adverse effects, they do not appear to exacerbate the toxicity of existing therapies, distinguishing them from other TLR agents that have been withdrawn from trials. The adoption of adaptive trial designs may optimize the evaluation of TLR agonists' efficacy and safety, enabling more efficient patient selection and treatment response assessment in oncology. The correlation between the anti-tumor effects of TLR agonists and the enhancement of dendritic cell and lymphocyte proliferation suggests their potential as clinical activity biomarkers, with ongoing studies expected to yield comprehensive efficacy and safety data for TLR agonists aimed at solid tumor treatment.

Author details

Mohammed AW. Almorish[1*] and Ali A. Alyahawi[2]

1 Department of Hematology, Faculty of Medicine and Health Sciences, Sana'a University, Sana'a, Yemen

2 Department of Clinical Pharmacy, Faculty of Clinical Pharmacy, 21 September University, Sana'a, Yemen

*Address all correspondence to: m.almorish@su.edu.ye; almorish70@gmail.com

References

[1] Cancer. World Health Organization. Available from: https://www.who.int/news-room/fact-sheets/detail/cancer. [Accessed: September 1, 2024]

[2] Risk Factors for Cancer—National Cancer Institute. Available from: https://www.cancer.gov/about-cancer/causes-prevention/risk [Accessed: September 1, 2024]

[3] Cancer Fact Sheet. World Heal Organ. Available from: https://www.who.int/newsroom/fact-sheets/detail/cancer [Accessed: September 1, 2024]

[4] Akira S, Uematsu S, Takeuchi O. Pathogen recognition and innate immunity. Cell. 2006;**124**:783-801. DOI: 10.1016/j.cell.2006.02.015

[5] Mukherjee S, Karmakar S, Babu SPS. TLR2 and TLR4 mediated host immune responses in major infectious diseases: A review. The Brazilian Journal of Infectious Diseases. 2016;**20**:193-204. DOI: 10.1016/j.bjid.2015.10.011

[6] Mukherjee S, Huda S, Sinha Babu SP. Toll-like receptor polymorphism in host immune response to infectious diseases: A review. Scandinavian Journal of Immunology. 2019;**90**:e12771. DOI: 10.1111/sji.12771

[7] Patra R, Das NC, Mukherjee S. Toll-like receptors (TLRs) as therapeutic targets for treating SARS-coV-2: An immunobiological perspective. Advances in Experimental Medicine and Biology. 2021;**1352**:87-109. DOI: 10.1007/978-3-030-85109-5_610. Behzadi E, Behzadi P. The role of toll-like receptors (TLRs) in urinary tract infections (UTIs). Cent Eur J Urol (2016) 69:404-10. doi: 10.5173/ceju.2016.871

[8] Behzadi P, Garcıa-Perdomo HA, Karpinski TM. Toll-like receptors: General molecular and structural biology. Journal of Immunology Research. 2021;**2021**:9914854. DOI: 10.1155/2021/9914854

[9] Mukherjee S, Karnam A, Das M, Babu SPS, Bayry J. *Wuchereria bancrofti* filaria activates human dendritic cells and polarizes T helper 1 and regulatory T cells via tolllike receptor 4. Communications Biology. 2019;**2**:1-11. DOI: 10.1038/s42003-019-0392-8

[10] Mukherjee S, Mukherjee S, Maiti TK, Bhattacharya S, Sinha Babu SP. A novel ligand of toll-like receptor 4 from the sheath of *Wuchereria bancrofti* microfilaria induces proinflammatory response in macrophages. The Journal of Infectious Diseases. 2017;**215**:954-965. DOI: 10.1093/infdis/jix067

[11] Yang Y, Li H, Fotopoulou C, Cunnea P, Zhao X. Toll-like receptor targeted anti-tumor therapies: Advances and challenges. Frontiers in Immunology. 2022;**13**:1049340. DOI: 10.3389/fimmu.2022.1049340

[12] Mukherjee S, Patra R, Behzadi P, Masotti A, Paolini A, Sarshar M. Toll-like receptor-guided therapeutic intervention of human cancers: Molecular and immunological perspectives. Frontiers in Immunology. 2023;**14**:1244345. DOI: 10.3389/fimmu.2023.1244345

[13] Kawai T, Ikegawa M, Ori D, Akira S. Decoding toll-like receptors: Recent insights and perspectives in innate immunity. Immunity. 2024;**57**(4):649-673. DOI: 10.1016/j.immuni.2024.03.004

[14] Deguine J, Barton GM. MyD88: A central player in innate immune

signaling. F1000Prime Rep. 2014;**6**:97. DOI: 10.12703/P6-97

[15] Chen L, Zheng L, Chen P, Liang G. Myeloid differentiation primary response protein 88 (MyD88): The central hub of TLR/IL-1R signaling. Journal of Medicinal Chemistry. 2020;**63**:13316-13329. DOI: 10.1021/acs.jmedchem.0c00884

[16] Wang L, Yu K, Zhang X, Yu S. Dual functional roles of the MyD88 signaling in colorectal cancer development. Biomedicine & Pharmacotherapy. 2018;**107**:177-184. DOI: 10.1016/j.biopha.2018.07.139

[17] Javaid N, Choi S. Toll-like receptors from the perspective of cancer treatment. Cancers (Basel). 2020;**12**:297

[18] Hasnat S et al. The prognostic value of toll-like receptors in head and neck squamous cell carcinoma: A systematic review and meta-analysis. International Journal of Molecular Sciences. 2020;**21**:7255

[19] Shi M et al. Application potential of toll-like receptors in cancer immunotherapy: Systematic review. Medicine (Baltimore). 2016;**95**:e3951

[20] Huang B et al. TLR signaling by tumor and immune cells: A double-edged sword. Oncogene. 2008;**27**:218-224

[21] Nishii N et al. Systemic administration of a TLR7 agonist attenuates regulatory T cells by dendritic cell modification and overcomes resistance to PD-L1 blockade therapy. Oncotarget. 2018;**9**:13301-13312

[22] Jensen SS et al. Systemic TLR7/8 micelles trigger a novel and potent anti-tumor response by strong recruitment of neutrophils leading to massive tumor cell killing. Journal of Clinical Oncology. 2022;**40**:2576-2576

[23] Ota Y et al. Novel intravenous injectable TLR7 agonist, DSP-0509, synergistically enhanced antitumor immune responses in combination with anti-PD-1 antibody [abstract]. In: Proceedings of the American Association for Cancer Research Annual Meeting 2018. Philadelphia (PA): AACR; 2018 Apr 14-18; Chicago, IL Cancer Res 2018;78: Abstract nr 4726

[24] Smith M et al. Trial watch: Toll-like receptor agonists in cancer immunotherapy. Oncoimmunology. 2018;**7**:e1526250

[25] Urban-Wojciuk Z et al. The role of TLRs in anti-cancer immunity and tumor rejection. Frontiers in Immunology. 2019;**10**:2388

[26] De Becker G et al. The adjuvant monophosphoryl lipid a increases the function of antigen-presenting cells. International Immunology. 2000;**12**:807-815

[27] Morton DL, Eilber FR, Holmes EC, Hunt JS, Ketcham AS, Silverstein MJ, et al. BCG immunotherapy of malignant melanoma: Summary of a seven-year experience. Annals of Surgery. 1974;**180**(4):635-643. DOI: 10.1097/00000658-197410000-00029

[28] Silverstein MJ, DeKernion J, Morton DL. Malignant melanoma metastatic to the bladder. Regression following intratumor injection of BCG vaccine. JAMA. 1974;**229**(6):688. DOI: 10.1001/jama.1974.03230440046032

[29] Morton DL, Mozzillo N, Thompson JF, Kelley MC, Faries M, Wagner J, et al. An international, randomized, phase III trial of bacillus Calmette-Guerin (BCG) plus allogeneic melanoma vaccine (MCV) or placebo

after complete resection of melanoma metastatic to regional or distant sites. Journal of Clinical Oncology. 2007;**25**(18_suppl):8508. DOI: 10.1200/jco.2007.25.18_suppl.8508

[30] Vermorken JB, Claessen AM, van Tinteren H, Gall HE, Ezinga R, Meijer S, et al. Active specific immunotherapy for stage II and stage III human colon cancer: A randomised trial. Lancet. 1999;**353**(9150):345-350. DOI: 10.1016/S0140-6736 (98)07186-4

[31] Uyl-de Groot CA, Vermorken JB, Hanna MG Jr, Verboom P, Groot MT, Bonsel GJ, et al. Immunotherapy with autologous tumor cell-BCG vaccine in patients with colon cancer: A prospective study of medical and economic benefits. Vaccine. 2005;**23**(17-18):2379-2387. DOI: 10.1016/j.vaccine.2005.01.015

[32] D'Agostini C, Pica F, Febbraro G, Grelli S, Chiavaroli C, Garaci E. Antitumour effect of OM-174 and cyclophosphamide on murine B16 melanoma in different experimental conditions. International Immunopharmacology. 2005;**5**(7-8):1205-1212. DOI: 10.1016/j.intimp.2005.02.013

[33] Kroemer G, Zitvogel L, Galluzzi L. Victories and deceptions in tumor immunology: Stimuvax(®). Oncoimmunology. 2013;**2**(1):e23687. DOI: 10.4161/onci.23687

[34] Brichard VG, Lejeune D. GSK's antigen-specific cancer immunotherapy programme: Pilot results leading to phase III clinical development. Vaccine. 2007;**25**(Suppl 2):B61-B71. DOI: 10.1016/j.vaccine.2007.06.038

[35] Bhatia S, Miller NJ, Lu H, Longino NV, Ibrani D, Shinohara MM, et al. Intratumoral G100, a TLR4 agonist, induces antitumor immune responses and tumor regression in patients with merkel cell carcinoma. Clinical Cancer Research. 2019;**25**(4):1185-1195. DOI: 10.1158/1078-0432.CCR-18-0469

[36] Lu H, Hewitt J, Jt M. Abstract 4885: Intratumoral injection of G100 (TLR4 agonist glycopyranosyl lipid a) modulates tumor microenvironment and induces CD8 T cell-dependent, systemic anti-tumor immunity. Cancer Research. 2016;**76**(14_Supplement):4885. DOI: 10.1158/1538-7445.AM2016-4885

[37] Steeghs N et al. Manufacturing-dependent change in biological activity of the TLR4 agonist GSK1795091 and implications for lipid a analog development. Clinical and Translational Science. 2022;**00**:1-15

[38] Burdelya LG, Krivokrysenko VI, Tallant TC, Strom E, Gleiberman AS, Gupta D, et al. An agonist of toll-like receptor 5 has radioprotective activity in mouse and primate models. Science. 2008;**320**(5873):226-230. DOI: 10.1126/science.1154986

[39] Sfondrini L, Rossini A, Besusso D, Merlo A, Tagliabue E, Mènard S, et al. Antitumor activity of the TLR-5 ligand flagellin in mouse models of cancer. Journal of Immunology. 2006;**176**(11):6624-6630. DOI: 10.4049/jimmunol.176.11.6624

[40] Mett V, Komarova EA, Greene K, Bespalov I, Brackett C, Gillard B, et al. Mobilan: A recombinant adenovirus carrying toll-like receptor 5 self-activating cassette for cancer immunotherapy. Oncogene. 2018;**37**(4):439-449. DOI: 10.1038/onc.2017.34

[41] Cai Z, Sanchez A, Shi Z, Zhang T, Liu M, Zhang D. Activation of toll-like receptor 5 on breast cancer cells by flagellin suppresses cell

proliferation and tumor growth. Cancer Research. 2011;**71**(7):2466-2475. DOI: 10.1158/0008-5472.CAN-10-1993

[42] Bakhribah H et al. A phase I study of the toll-like receptor 5 (TLR5) agonist, entolimod in patients (pts) with advanced cancers. Journal of Clinical Oncology. 2015;**33**:3063

[43] Cleveland BioLabs. Cleveland BioLabs announces start of colorectal cancer study of entolimod in Russian Federation [press release]. 2016. Available from: https://novamedica.com/media/theme_news/p/4199-cleveland-biolabs-announces-start-of-colorectal-cancer-study-of-entolimod-in-russian-federation [Accessed: September 1, 2024]

[44] Mett V, Kurnasov OV, Bespalov IA, Molodtsov I, Brackett CM, Burdelya LG, et al. A deimmunized and pharmacologically optimized toll-like receptor 5 agonist for therapeutic applications. Communications Biology. 2021;**4**(1):466. DOI: 10.1038/s42003-021-01978-6

[45] Gonzalez C, Williamson S, Gammon ST, et al. TLR5 agonists enhance anti-tumor immunity and overcome resistance to immune checkpoint therapy. Communications Biology. 2023;**6**:31. DOI: 10.1038/s42003-022-04403-8

[46] Alexopoulou L, Holt AC, Medzhitov R, Flavell RA. Recognition of doublestranded RNA and activation of NF-kappaB by toll-like receptor 3. Nature. 2001;**413**(6857):732-738. DOI: 10.1038/35099560

[47] Kato H, Takeuchi O, Mikamo-Satoh E, Hirai R, Kawai T, Matsushita K, et al. Length-dependent recognition of double-stranded ribonucleic acids by retinoic acidinducible gene-I and melanoma differentiation-associated gene 5. The Journal of Experimental Medicine. 2008;**205**(7):1601-1610. DOI: 10.1084/jem.20080091

[48] Datta SK, Redecke V, Prilliman KR, Takabayashi K, Corr M, Tallant T, et al. A subset of toll-like receptor ligands induces cross-presentation by bone marrow-derived dendritic cells1. Journal of Immunology. 2003;**170**(8):4102-4110. DOI: 10.4049/jimmunol.170.8.4102

[49] Isakoff SJ, Tolaney SM, Tung NM, Adams S, Soliman HH, Brachtel EF, et al. A phase 1b study of safety and immune response to PVX-410 vaccine alone and in combination with durvalumab (MEDI4736) in HLA-A2+ patients following adjuvant therapy for stage 2/3 triple negative breast cancer. Journal of Clinical Oncology. 2017;**35**(15_suppl):TPS1126-TPS1TPS. DOI: 10.1200/JCO.2017.35.15_suppl.TPS1126

[50] Karki NR, Bano K, Ramses S, Nayak A. A phase II trial of pembrolizumab and poly-ICLC in patients with metastatic mismatch repair-proficient colon cancer. Journal of Clinical Oncology. 2021;**39**(15_suppl):e15552–e. DOI: 10.1200/JCO.2021.39.15_suppl.e15552

[51] Matijevic Glavan T, Pavelic J. The exploitation of toll-like receptor 3 signaling in cancer therapy. Current Pharmaceutical Design. 2014;**20**(42):6555-6564. DOI: 10.2174/1381612820666140826153347

[52] Lee S-H, Choi Y-H, Kang SM, Lee M-G, Debin A, Perouzel E, et al. The defined TLR3 agonist, nexavant, exhibits anti-cancer efficacy and potentiates anti-PD-1 antibody therapy by enhancing immune cell infiltration. Cancers. 2023;**15**(24):5752. DOI: 10.3390/cancers15245752

[53] Radolec MOB, Vlad A, Vlad A, Vlad A, Vlad A, Vlad A, et al. Systemic

immune checkpoint blockade and intraperitoneal chemo-immunotherapy in recurrent ovarian cancer: An interim analysis. Gynecologic Oncology. 2022;**166**:S165-S166. DOI: 10.1016/S0090-8258(22)01540-2

[54] Navabi H, Jasani B, Reece A, Clayton A, Tabi Z, Donninger C, et al. A clinical grade poly I:C-analogue (Ampligen) promotes optimal DC maturation and Th1-type T cell responses of healthy donors and cancer patients in vitro. Vaccine. 2009;**27**(1):107-115. DOI: 10.1016/j.vaccine.2008.10.024

[55] Gandhi SOM, Ford C, Slomba R, Quinn M, O'Connor T, Levine E, et al. Safety and efficacy of de-escalated neoadjuvant Chemoimmunotherapy of triple negative breast cancer (TNBC) using chemokine-modulating regimen (rintatolimod, IFN-α2b, celecoxib). Journal of ImmunoTherapy of Cancer. 2022;**2022**:5

[56] Sheybani ND, Witter AR, Thim EA, Yagita H, Bullock TNJ, Price RJ. Combination of thermally ablative focused ultrasound with gemcitabine controls breast cancer via adaptive immunity. Journal for Immunotherapy of Cancer. 2020;**2020**:8

[57] Le Naour J, Kroemer G. Trial watch: Toll-like receptor ligands in cancer therapy. Oncoimmunology. 2023;**12**(1):2180237. DOI: 10.1080/2162402X.2023.2180237

[58] Marquez-Rodas I, Dalle S, Castanon E, Sanmamed MF, Arance AM, Cerezuela-Fuentes P, et al. Combination of radiomic and biomarker signatures as exploratoryobjective in a phase II trial with intratumoral BO-112 plus pembrolizumab for advanced melanoma. Journal of Clinical Oncology. 2021;**39**(15_suppl):9586. DOI: 10.1200/JCO.2021.39.15_suppl.TPS9586

[59] Rodas IM, Saiag P, LdlC M, Dutriaux C, Rodríguez-Moreno J, Robert C, et al. 961 preliminary results of a phase 2 study of intratumoral administration of BO-112 with pembrolizumab in patients with advanced melanoma that have progressive disease on anti-PD-1-based therapy. Journal of ImmunoTherapy of Cancer. 2021;**9**(Suppl 2):A1011-A10A2. DOI: 10.1136/jitc-2021-SITC2021.961

[60] Diebold SS, Kaisho T, Hemmi H, Akira S, Reis e Sousa C. Innate antiviral responses by means of TLR7-mediated recognition of single-stranded RNA. Science. 2004;**303**:1529-1531

[61] Patel GK, Goodwin R, Chawla M, Laidler P, Price PE, Finlay AY, et al. Imiquimod 5% cream monotherapy for cutaneous squamous cell carcinoma in situ (Bowen's disease): A randomized, double-blind, placebo-controlled trial. Journal of the American Academy of Dermatology. 2006;**54**(6):1025-1032

[62] Chakraborty S, Ye J, Wang H, Sun M, Zhang Y, Sang X, et al. Application of toll-like receptors (TLRs) and their agonists in cancer vaccines and immunotherapy. Frontiers in Immunology. 2023;**14**:1227833. DOI: 10.3389/fimmu.2023.1227833

[63] Hu Y et al. Safety, pharmacokinetics and pharmacodynamics of TQ-A3334, an oral toll-like receptor 7 agonist in healthy individuals. Expert Opinion on Investigational Drugs. 2021;**30**:1-7

[64] Zuo X, Cheng Q, Wang Z, Liu J, Wanjun L, Guannan W, et al. A novel oral TLR7 agonist orchestrates immune response and synergizes with PD-L1 blockade via type I IFN pathway in lung cancer. International Immunopharmacology. 2024;**137**:112478. DOI: 10.1016/j.intimp.2024.112478

[65] Curigliano et al. Phase I study of LHC165 ± spartalizumab (PDR001) in patients (pts) with advanced solid tumors. Cancer Research. 2021;**81**:CT103. DOI: 10.1158/1538-7445.AM2021-CT103

[66] Curigliano G, Jimenez MM, Shimizu T, Keam B, Meric-Bernstam F, Rutten A, et al. A phase I trial of LHC165 single agent and in combination with spartalizumab in patients with advanced solid malignancies. ESMO open. 2024;**9**(8):103643. DOI: 10.1016/j.esmoop.2024.103643

[67] Symeonides S, Mahalingam D, Chae YK, et al. 525 Preliminary safety, PK/PD and efficacy results from a first-in-human phase I/IIa clinical trial of BNT411, a systemic Toll-like receptor 7 agonist in patients with solid tumors. Journal for Immuno Therapy of Cancer 2021;**9**(Suppl 2):A555-A555. DOI: 10.1136/jitc-2021-SITC2021.525

[68] Janku F, Han SW, Doi T, Amatu A, Ajani JA, Kuboki Y, et al. Preclinical characterization and phase I study of an anti-HER2-TLR7 immune-stimulator antibody conjugate in patients with HER2+ malignancies. Cancer Immunology Research. 2022;**10**(12):1441-1461. DOI: 10.1158/2326-6066.CIR-21-0722

[69] Janku F, Doi T, Ajani J, Kuboki Y, Mahling P, Subramanian K, et al. A first in-human, multicenter,open-label, dose-finding phase 1 study of the immune stimulator antibody conjugate NJH395 in patients with nonbreast HER2+advanced malignancies. Journal for Immunotherapy of Cancer. 2020;**8**(Suppl 3):A230. DOI: 10.1136/jitc-2020-SITC2020.0378

[70] Rolfo C, Giovannetti E, Martinez P, McCue S, Naing A. Applications and clinical trial landscape using toll-like receptor agonists to reduce the toll of cancer. npj Precision Oncology. 2023;**7**(1):26. DOI: 10.1038/s41698-023-00364-1

[71] Patel M et al. BDB001, a toll-like receptor 7 and 8 (TLR7/8) agonist, can be safely administered intravenously and shows clinical responses in advanced solid tumors. Journal for Immunotherapy of Cancer. 2020;**8**:A199

[72] Patel MR et al. BDB001, an intravenously administered toll-like receptor 7 and 8 (TLR7/8) agonist, in combination with pembrolizumab in advanced solid tumors: Phase 1 safety and efficacy results. Journal of Clinical Oncology. 2021;**39**:2512

[73] Sharma M et al. Phase 1/2 study of novel HER2-targeting, TLR7/8 immune stimulating antibody conjugate (ISAC) BDC-1001 with or without immune checkpoint inhibitor in patients with advanced HER2-expressing solid tumors. Journal for Immunotherapy of Cancer. 2020;**8**:A224

[74] Crd SM, Hanna GJ, Li BT, Moore KN, Pegram MD, Rasco DW, et al. Preliminary results from a phase 1/2 study of BDC-1001, a novel HER2 targeting TLR7/8 immune-stimulating antibody conjugate (ISAC), in patients (pts) with advanced HER2-expressing solid tumors. Journal of Clinical Oncology. 2021;**39**(15):2549

[75] Eigentler T et al. A phase I dose-escalation and expansion study of intratumoral CV8102 as single-agent or in combination with anti-PD-1 antibodies in patients with advanced solid tumors. Journal of Clinical Oncology. 2020;**38**:3096

[76] Löffler MW, Gori S, Izzo F, Mayer-Mokler A, Ascierto PA, Königsrainer A, et al. Phase I/II multicenter trial of a novel therapeutic

cancer vaccine, HepaVac-101, for hepatocellular carcinoma. Clinical Cancer Research: An Official Journal of the American Association for Cancer Research. 2022;**28**(12):2555-2566. DOI: 10.1158/1078-0432.CCR-21-4424

[77] Zúñiga LA et al. Intratumoral delivery of TransCon™ TLR7/8 agonist promotes sustained anti-tumor activity and local immune cell activation while minimizing systemic cytokine induction. Cancer Cell International. 2022;**22**:286. DOI: 10.1186/s12935-022-02708-6

[78] Ascendis Pharma. Ascendis Pharma A/S virtual R&D program update highlights continued development across R&D pipeline [press release]. 2021. Available from: https://investors.ascendispharma.com/node/11076/pdf [Accessed: September 1, 2024]

[79] Emens L, Beeram M, Hamilton E, Piha-Paul S, Odegard V, Hamke S, et al. A phase 1/1b study of SBT6050, a HER2-directed monoclonal antibody conjugated to a toll-like receptor 8 agonist, in subjects with advanced HER2-expressing solid tumors. Journal of ImmunoTherapy of Cancer. 2020;**8**:317

[80] Klempner SJBM, Sabanathan D, Chan A, Hamilton E, Loi S, Oh D, et al. Interim results from phase 1/1b study of SBT6050 alone or In combination with pembrolizumab in advanced or metastatic HER2-expressing solid tumors. Annals Oncology. 2021;**32**:S450. DOI: 10.1016/j.annonc. 2021.08.491

[81] Comeau MR, Metz H, Stevens B, Winship D, Brevik J, Rhodehamel M, et al. Abstract 1858: SBT6290, a systemically administered Nectin4-directed TLR8 ImmunoTAC™ product candidate, is designed for tumor-localized activation of myeloid cells. Cancer Research. 2021;**81**(13_Supplement):1858. DOI: 10.1158/1538-7445.AM2021-1858

[82] Vollmer J et al. Characterization of three CpG oligodeoxynucleotide classes with distinct immunostimulatory activities. European Journal of Immunology. 2004;**34**:251-262

[83] Karapetyan L, Luke JJ, Davar D. Toll-like receptor 9 agonists in cancer. Oncotargets and Therapy. 2020;**13**:10039-10060. DOI: 10.2147/OTT.S247050

[84] Mologen AG. MOLOGEN AG Announces Top Line Data of Pivotal IMPALA Study In metastatic Colorectal Cancer [Press Release]. Berlin: MOLOGEN AG; 2019. Available from: https://bwnews.pr/2MFs9MR [Accessed: September 1, 2024]

[85] Schmoll HJ et al. Maintenance treatment with the immunomodulator MGN1703, a toll-like receptor 9 (TLR9) agonist, in patients with metastatic colorectal carcinoma and disease control after chemotherapy: A randomised, double-blind, placebo-controlled trial. Journal of Cancer Research and Clinical Oncology. 2014;**140**:1615-1624

[86] Shakoora S, Andrew V, Laura R, et al. Abstract 6666: Evaluation of the complexity of the immune response to CMP-001, a TLR9 agonist. Cancer Research. 2020;**80**(16 Suppl):6666. DOI: 10.1158/1538-7445.AM2020-6666

[87] Milhem M et al. Intratumoral injection of CMP-001, a toll-like receptor 9 (TLR9) agonist, in combination with pembrolizumab reversed programmed death receptor 1 (PD-1) blockade resistance in advanced melanoma. Journal for Immunotherapy of Cancer. 2020;**8**:A186-A187

[88] Davar D et al. Phase II trial of neoadjuvant nivolumab (Nivo) and intra-tumoral (IT) CMP-001 in high-risk

resectable melanoma (neo-C-Nivo): Final results. Journal for Immunotherapy of Cancer. 2020;**8**:A185-A186

[89] Negrao M et al. TLR9 agonist CMP-001 plus atezolizumab +/− radiation therapy in patients with PD-1 blockade resistant advanced NSCLC. Journal of Thoracic Oncology. 2021;**16**:S196

[90] Milhem MM et al. Phase 1b/2, open label, multicenter, study of the combination of SD-101 and pembrolizumab in patients with advanced melanoma who are naïve to anti-PD-1 therapy. Journal of Clinical Oncology. 2019;**37**:9534

[91] Dynavax. Overall response rate of 76% in advanced melanoma patients with Dynavax's SD-101 in combination with KEYTRUDA® (pembrolizumab); data presented today at the 2019 ASCO annual meeting [press release]. Available from: https://investors.dynavax.com/news-releases/news-release-details/overallresponse-rate-76-advanced-melanoma-patients-dynavaxs-sd. [Accessed: September 1, 2024]

[92] Cohen E. Intralesional SD-101 in combination with pembrolizumab in anti-PD-1 treatment-naïve head and neck squamous cell carcinoma: Results from a multicenter, phase II trial. Clinical Cancer Research. 2022;**28**:1157-1166

[93] O'Day S et al. Safety and preliminary efficacy of intratumoral cavrotolimod (AST- 008), a spherical nucleic acid TLR9 agonist, in combination with pembrolizumab in patients with advanced solid tumors. Journal for Immunotherapy of Cancer. 2020;**8**:A257-A258

[94] Milhem MM et al. Phase 1b/2 study of an intratumoral TLR9 agonist spherical nucleic acid (AST-008) and pembrolizumab: Evidence of immune activation. Cancer Research. 2020;**80**(16 Suppl):Abstract LB-140. DOI: 10.1158/1538-7445.AM2020-LB-140

[95] Haymaker C et al. Final results from ILLUMINATE-204, a phase I/II trial of intratumoral tilsotolimod in combination with ipilimumab in PD-1 inhibitor refractory advanced melanoma. Annals of Oncology. 2020;**31**:S672-S710

Section 3

Modulation of Innate Immunity in Organ Transplantation and Mitochondrial Dysfunction

Chapter 6

Understanding the Immunological Significance of Blood Groups in Organ Transplantation

B. Pushpa, R.A. Shanmugha Priya, Ushus S. Kumar and J. Saminathan

Abstract

This chapter investigates the relationship between blood groups and the immune system in the background of organ transplantation. It explores how blood group compatibility plays a serious role in determining the success of organ transplants and mitigating the risk of rejection. The chapter focuses on the underlying mechanisms that affect graft acceptance or rejection by looking at the immunological importance of blood types. It explores the complex interactions between antibodies, antigens, and the immune response and emphasizes how variations in blood type antigens may trigger the immunological reactions and affect the success of transplants. Furthermore, the clinical implications of blood group matching in organ transplantation are also highlighted in this chapter. It also discusses emerging advancements in immunogenetics and immunosuppressive therapies that aim to overcome the immunological challenges associated with blood group disparities. Overall. The chapter serves as a valuable resource for healthcare professionals and researchers to facilitate improved matching strategies and enhanced outcomes in the field of transplantation medicine.

Keywords: blood groups, immune system, organ transplantation, blood group compatibility, risk of rejection, blood types

1. Introduction

The study aims to examine the influence of blood groups on the outcomes of organ transplantation [1]. By examining how different blood groups interact with the immune system, this research seeks to uncover the potential impact on graft acceptance, rejection rates, and overall success of transplantation procedures. Through a comprehensive understanding of these immunological interactions, the study aims to provide insights that could guide improved strategies for organ compatibility assessment and enhance transplantation outcomes [2]. Organ transplantation stands as a pinnacle of modern medical achievement, offering a transformative solution for individuals facing life-threatening organ failure. This complex procedure involves replacing a malfunctioning or injured organ with a vigorous one from a donor, often providing patients with renewed vitality and extended life. The significance of organ

IntechOpen

transplantation lies in its ability to save lives, restore function, and enhance the quality of life for recipients who might otherwise be confined to a life of medical intervention. As medical knowledge and surgical techniques continue to advance, organ transplantation has evolved from an experimental endeavor to a well-established medical practice, making a profound impact on the lives of countless individuals and their families. The significance of organ transplantation reaches far beyond medical treatment. It embodies the potential to transform a patient's existence from one of suffering and limitations to a life of renewed vitality [3]. Transplant recipients often experience not only physical relief but also a newfound sense of purpose as they resume everyday activities, pursue careers, and engage in hobbies that were once distant dreams. This restoration of functionality has a cascading effect on their mental and emotional well-being, illustrating how organ transplantation is more than just a medical procedure; it's a gateway to a second chance at life.

The impact of organ transplantation extends beyond individual patients, influencing society and healthcare systems [4]. While the procedure comes with initial costs, the long-term benefits are compelling. Successful transplants reduce the need for ongoing treatments like dialysis or extended hospital stays, relieving the burden on healthcare resources. Furthermore, recipients' return to active lives contributes to a stronger workforce and reduced strain on social services. This underscores how organ transplantation is not only a medical triumph but also an avenue toward more efficient and sustainable healthcare practices [5]. However, the field of organ transplantation is not without its challenges. Ethical considerations surrounding organ procurement, distribution, and the use of living donors require careful navigation. As medical science evolves, research continues to explore regenerative medicine, innovative transplantation techniques, and personalized approaches. These endeavors offer hope for overcoming existing limitations, addressing organ shortages, and ultimately improving the success rates and accessibility of organ transplantation. Organ transplantation serves as a testament to human ingenuity, medical progress, and the unwavering pursuit of life-enhancing solutions in the realm of modern medicine. Moreover, blood groups play a pivotal role in determining the compatibility of organ transplantation [6]. These groups, categorized as A, B, AB, and O, are well-defined by explicit antigens existing on the surface of red blood cells. Blood group compatibility is crucial in transplantation to mitigate potential immunological challenges. When an organ is transplanted, the immune system of the donor can identify the antigens on the donor's cells as distant, activating an immune reaction that may lead to graft rejection.

The compatibility of blood groups among the donor and recipient is fundamental to the success of an organ transplant [7]. Mismatched blood groups can evoke an immune response categorized by the production of antibodies alongside the foreign antigens. This response can lead to hyperacute rejection, a speedy and stark form of rejection that happens within minutes to hours afterwards transplantation. The antibodies can activate complement proteins, causing extensive damage to the transplanted organ's blood vessels and ultimately resulting in organ failure. Incompatibility in blood groups can also lead to acute and chronic rejection over time, as the immune system continuously targets the foreign antigens [8]. Understanding the immunological challenges posed by blood group disparities is essential to devising effective transplant strategies. Immunosuppressive therapies are employed to dampen the immune response and prevent rejection. However, managing immunosuppression while maintaining a functioning immune system poses a delicate balance, as excessive suppression can increase susceptibility to infections and other complications. Additionally, advancements in transplant techniques, such as cross matching and tissue typing, have been crucial in assessing compatibility and minimizing the risk of rejection. The intricate interplay between blood group compatibility and the immune response highlights the necessity of meticulous donor-recipient matching and underscores the ongoing research efforts to refine transplantation procedures and enhance long-term graft survival.

The key contributions of this paper is given as follows:

- The research builds light on how different blood groups impact the compatibility between donors and recipients in organ transplantation.
- By elucidating the complex immunological interactions involved, it provides valuable insights for refining compatibility assessments, ultimately leading to better organ matching and reduced risk of rejection.
- The research tailors immunosuppressive strategies and innovative desensitization techniques that mitigate the risk of immune responses, particularly those stemming from blood group incompatibilities.
- The research prepares healthcare professionals with crucial information to make informed decisions regarding organ allocation and transplantation priority.
- The research underscores the importance of ongoing investigations into blood group immunology, stimulating further research and innovation in the field of organ transplantation.

2. Blood groups and compatibility

The ABO and RhD blood group systems are two of the most well-known and clinically significant blood group systems that play a crucial role in blood compatibility, organ transplantation, and pregnancy [9]. These systems are strong-minded by particular antigens that are existing on the surface of red blood cells.

2.1 ABO and RhD blood group system

The ABO blood group system orders blood into four main groups: A, B, AB, and O, grounded on the occurrence or nonappearance of two antigens: A and B antigens [10]. These antigens are glycoproteins located on the surface of red blood cells. The A antigen is contemporary in blood type A, the B antigen is present in blood type B, both antigens are existing in blood type AB, and neither antigen is present in blood type O. Additionally, individuals possess antibodies compared to the antigens they lack. For example, a person with blood type A has anti-B antibodies, and a person with blood type B has anti-A antibodies. Blood type AB individuals do not produce these antibodies, while blood type O entities yield both anti-A and anti-B antibodies. This antigen-antibody interaction is important in blood transfusions to prevent adverse reactions. It also produces a risk known as Graft rejection. And it is caused due to ABO incompatibility in organ transplantation. Moreover, it potentially leading to graft failure and adverse patient outcomes. ABO-incompatible transplants can trigger severe immune responses, such as hyperacute rejection, driven by preformed antibodies targeting non-self ABO antigens. These immune reactions result in rapid damage to the transplanted organ, compromising its function and often necessitating emergency retransplantation.

2.2 RhD blood group system

The RhD blood group system, often referred to as the Rh factor or Rh antigen, focuses on the occurrence or nonappearance of the RhD antigen on the surface of red blood cells [11]. Individuals having this antigen are Rh-positive (e.g., A+, B+), while those lacking the antigen are Rh-negative (e.g., A−, B−). The RhD system is particularly important during pregnancy. An Rh-negative mother booming an Rh-positive fetus may progress antibodies alongside the RhD antigen if their blood mixes, potentially leading to hemolytic disease of the newborn (HDN) in subsequent pregnancies. To prevent HDN, Rh-negative pregnant women may receive Rh immunoglobulin (RhIg) to prevent antibody formation. These blood group systems hold critical clinical significance in blood transfusions and organ transplantation. ABO compatibility is essential to prevent adverse reactions during blood transfusions, while Rh compatibility is crucial for preventing sensitization in cases of Rh-negative individuals receiving Rh-positive blood. In organ transplantation, matching blood groups between donors and recipients is a vital consideration to minimize the risk of graft rejection due to immune responses against unmatched antigens.

Incompatibility in the Rh system can lead to the production of anti-Rh antibodies in Rh-negative individuals if they are exposed to Rh-positive blood. This is particularly relevant during pregnancy when an Rh-negative mother transfers an Rh-positive fetus. **Figure 1** depicts the ABO-RhD diagram.

2.3 Supplementary blood group systems

In addition to the ABO and RhD blood group systems, there are several other important blood group antigen systems that play a crucial role in organ transplantation, immune responses, and overall compatibility [12]. Two notable systems are the Human Leukocyte Antigen (HLA) system and the Major Histocompatibility Complex (MHC) play an important role in transplant immunology.

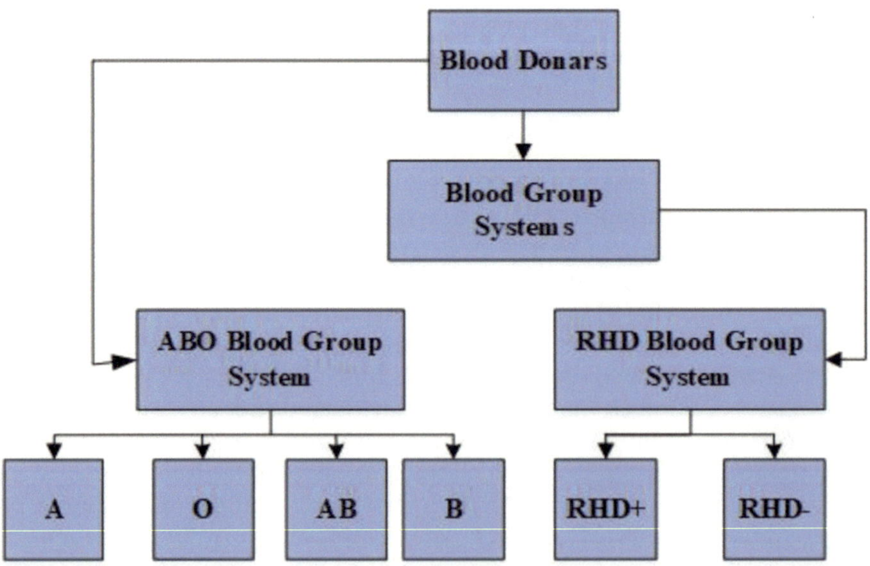

Figure 1.
ABO-RHD diagram.

2.3.1 Human leukocyte antigen (HLA) system

The HLA system, also known as the human MHC (Major Histocompatibility Complex), is a extremely diverse group of DNAs positioned on chromosome 6. HLA molecules play a pivotal role in the immune system by presenting antigens to T cells, which regulate immune responses [13]. HLA particles are established on the surface of various cells, including immune cells and transplantable tissues. Two main classes of HLA are: HLA class I (HLA-A, HLA-B, and HLA-C) and HLA class II (HLA-DR, HLA-DP, and HLA-DQ). In organ transplantation, HLA compatibility is crucial for graft survival. Mismatched HLA antigens can trigger immune responses, leading to acute or chronic rejection of the transplanted organ. The immune system distinguishes the foreign HLA antigens as non-self and can mount an immune response against the transplanted tissue. To enhance organ transplant success, HLA matching between the donor and recipient is carefully considered. **Figure 2** depicts the diagrammatic representation of HLA.

2.3.2 Major histocompatibility complex (MHC)

The Major Histocompatibility Complex (MHC), is also acknowledged as the Human Leukocyte Antigen (HLA) structure in humans and also it is also considered as a cluster of genetic factor that scramble cell surface proteins responsible for presenting antigens to the immune system [14]. The MHC is a dangerous constituent of the immune response and plays a central part in immune recognition, self-versus-non-self-discrimination, and immune system regulation. The MHC is separated into two main sessions: MHC class I and MHC class II.

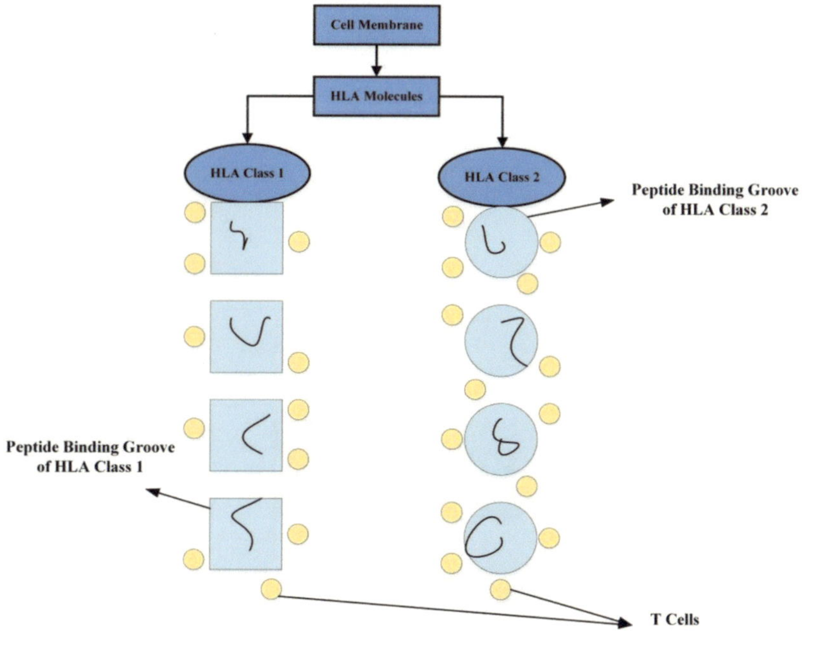

Figure 2.
Diagrammatic representation of HLA.

2.3.2.1 MHC class I

MHC class I particles are initiated on the surface of nearly all nucleated cells in the body [15]. They play a crucial role in bestowing antigens consequent from within the cell, such as viral or intracellular bacterial proteins, to cytotoxic T cells (CD8+ T cells). This presentation helps the immune system identify and destroy infected or abnormal cells. MHC class I particles comprise of a transmembrane heavy chain, light chain and a small protein fragment called a peptide, which is derived from the internal antigens.

2.3.2.2 MHC class II

MHC class II particles are primarily created on the exterior of antigen-presenting cells, like dendritic cells, macrophages, and B cells [16]. These molecules present antigens consequents from extracellular pathogens, like bacteria and fungi, to helper T cells (CD4+ T cells). This interaction is crucial for activating and regulating immune responses. MHC class II molecules also consist of a transmembrane heavy chain and a peptide fragment, but they interact with different types of T cells compared to MHC class I. **Figure 3** depicts the diagrammatic representation of MHC.

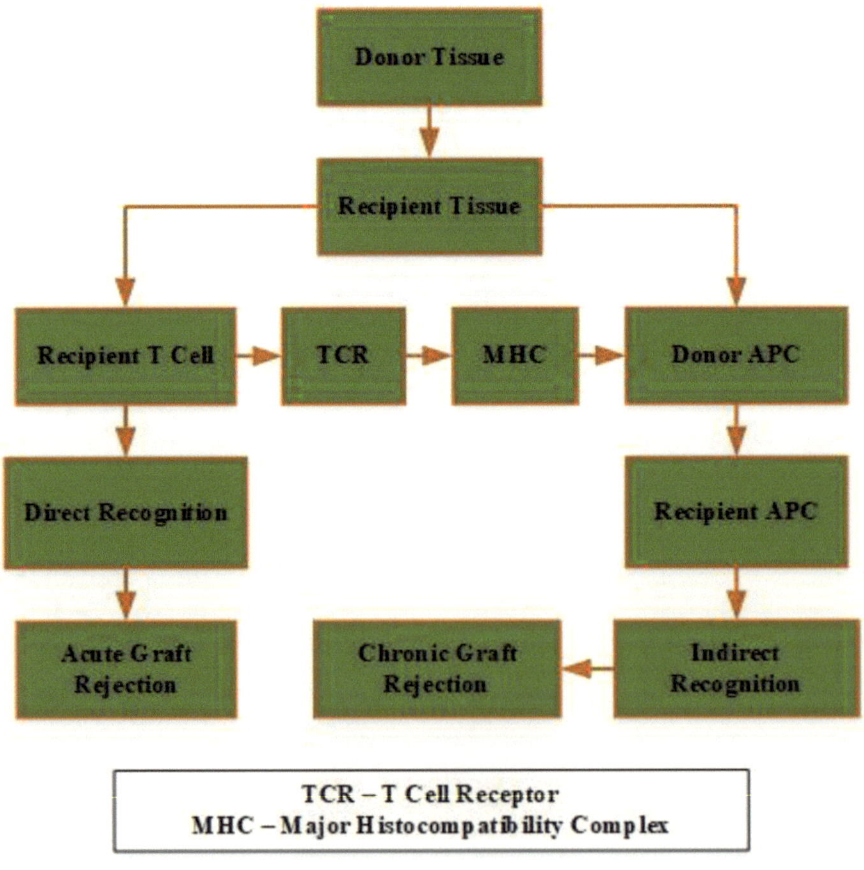

Figure 3.
Diagrammatic representation of MHC.

2.4 Cross matching

Cross matching is a pivotal pre-transplantation laboratory test that evaluates the compatibility between a recipient's immune system and a potential organ donor. It encompasses both direct and indirect methods to recognize antibodies in the recipient's serum that could respond against antigens on the donor's tissue. In direct cross matching, the recipient's antibodies are tested against the donor's cells, while in indirect cross matching, recipient cell is verified in contrast to donor serum. A positive cross match indicates potential incompatibility, signaling a risk of immune-mediated rejection and hyperacute rejection [17]. Strategies like desensitization, plasmapheresis, intravenous immunoglobulin (IVIG), and immunosuppressive medications can be employed to mitigate the risk in cases of positive cross matches. By preventing adverse immune reactions, cross matching enhances the success of organ transplantation and contributes to improved recipient outcomes. In blood transfusions, non-ABO antigens, such as those from the Rh and other blood group systems, can trigger immune responses if the recipient's immune system identifies these antigens as foreign. This can lead to hemolysis, transfusion reactions, and other adverse effects. By minimizing immune responses against these antigens, blood transfusions can be carried out safely and effectively, ensuring that the transfused blood components are compatible with the recipient's immune system. Minimizing immune responses against non-ABO antigens is of paramount importance in various medical contexts, particularly in blood transfusions and organ transplantation. While ABO compatibility is a critical consideration, the immune system's response to non-ABO antigens, particularly those were associated to the HLA system, can significantly impact the success of these medical procedures. Moreover, minimizing immune responses against non-ABO antigens is essential to avoid complications in treatments like bone marrow and stem cell transplantation. Mismatched HLA antigens can lead to graft-versus-host disease (GVHD), where immune cells from the transplanted tissue destroy the recipient's tissues.

3. Immunological basis of blood group compatibility

Blood group compatibility is founded on the complicated interaction among the immune system and the distinct antigens present on the surface of red blood cells [18]. The major blood group systems, such as ABO and Rh, are key determinants of compatibility in blood transfusions and organ transplants. The ABO system, for instance, is governed by the occurrence or nonappearance of A and B antigens, which are formed by glycosyltransferases encoded by the ABO gene. These antigens act as markers that are recognized by the immune system as either self or non-self. Incompatible blood transfusions can trigger an immune response as a consequence of the immune system's recognition of non-self-antigens. Individuals possess naturally occurring antibodies compared to the ABO antigens they lack. For instance, individuals with blood type A have anti-B antibodies, while those with blood type B have anti-A antibodies. In type O individuals, who lack both A and B antigens, both anti-A and anti-B antibodies are present. Upon exposure to non-self-antigens, these antibodies can drag to the distant antigens on transfused red blood cells, inducing agglutination and potential blockages within blood vessels, leading to serious complications. The immune basis of blood group compatibility extends to the Rh system as well. The Rh antigen, also recognized as the D antigen, is a critical determinant in Rh-positive and Rh-negative blood types. Rh-negative individuals can create antibodies in contrast to the Rh antigen if exposed to Rh-positive blood. This becomes particularly relevant for pregnant Rh-negative women bearing an Rh-positive fetus, as maternal antibodies can cross the placenta, potentially leading to hemolytic disease of the newborn.

3.1 Hyperacute rejection by anti-A and anti-B antibodies

Hyperacute rejection is a rapid and severe immune response that occurs in organ transplantation when the recipient's preformed antibodies react against antigens on the transplanted organ's vascular endothelium [19]. The presence of anti-A and anti-B antibodies can contribute to hyperacute rejection. When an organ from a donor with a different ABO blood type is transplanted into a recipient, the ABO antigens present on the surface of the transplanted organ's blood vessels can trigger an immediate immune response. This happens because the recipient's immune system identifies these ABO antigens as distant and targets them with the preformed antibodies that are specific to the antigens they lack. For example, if a blood type A individual obtains an organ from a blood type B donor, the recipient's immune system contains preformed anti-B antibodies. These antibodies can quickly drag to the B antigens on the transplanted organ's blood vessels. This binding triggers a series of events, including activation of complement proteins and recruitment of immune cells, which leads to inflammation, blood clot formation, and damage to the blood vessels and the organ itself. This process can occur within minutes to hours after transplantation, resulting in the failure of the transplanted organ.

The exploration of the immunological significance of blood groups in transplantation has yielded valuable insights, yet several promising areas for future research remain. Firstly, investigating the underlying mechanisms that drive hyperacute rejection due to ABO incompatibility could lead to more targeted interventions. Understanding the factors influencing the rapid activation of complement proteins and immune cells upon encountering non-self ABO antigens could potentially open avenues for developing therapies that mitigate this severe form of rejection. Also, delving into the complexities of the immune response against non-ABO antigens, such as those within the HLA system, offers an opportunity to enhance transplantation outcomes further. Research could focus on deciphering the intricacies of T cell recognition and activation in response to mismatched HLA antigens. This could lead to the development of personalized immunosuppressive strategies that dampen the immune response while preserving the overall immune function, thereby improving long-term graft survival.

Moreover, advancements in immunogenetics and molecular techniques also present exciting avenues. Investigating genetic variations that influence immune responses to blood group antigens could yield insights into individual susceptibility to rejection. This could pave the way for precision medicine approaches that tailor transplant protocols based on a recipient's genetic profile, enhancing compatibility and minimizing adverse reactions. Therefore, exploring the role of non-ABO antigens beyond direct graft rejection is an emerging research area. Investigating how these antigens influence the immune microenvironment post-transplantation and their potential impact on long-term graft health could lead to more comprehensive strategies for immunomodulation and graft preservation.

3.2 Character of preformed antibodies and supplement stimulation in graft damage

Preformed antibodies and supplement stimulation play critical roles in graft damage, particularly in the background of organ transplantation and autoimmune diseases [20]. These mechanisms contribute to hyperacute rejection in organ transplantation and can exacerbate tissue damage in autoimmune conditions. Preformed antibodies are immune molecules that have been previously generated in response to antigens encountered in previous infections or sensitization events. In the context of organ transplantation, preformed antibodies can identify distant antigens on the transplanted organ's surface. This acknowledgment generates a rapid and powerful immune response that can lead to graft damage. In hyperacute rejection, preformed antibodies specifically target the antigens present on the transplanted organ, initiating a cascade of immune reactions that include complement activation. Complement activation is a series of enzymatic reactions that involve a group of proteins called the supplement system. The supplement system can be stimulated through the classical, lectin, or alternate pathways. When preformed antibodies bind to antigens on the graft, they can trigger the classical conduit of supplement activation. This pointers to the sequential cleavage of complement proteins, ultimately resulting in the development of membrane attack complexes (MACs) that puncture the cell membranes of the target tissue or graft cells. This leads to cell lysis, inflammation, and tissue damage.

4. Impact on transplantation success

However, the extent of non-adherence to immunosuppressants varies among different categories of transplant recipients [21]. The findings reveal that kidney recipients exhibit the highest non-adherence prevalence, with a rate of 38 cases of100 patient per years (PPY). This rate surpasses that detected in heart recipients by more than two-fold and exceeds liver recipients by over five-fold. The lower rates in the latter groups could stem from the diverse practices across programs, possibly implementing more rigorous psychosocial criteria during the transplant candidate selection process compared to kidney candidates. Alternatively, the higher stakes of graft loss may contribute: while kidney recipients can resume dialysis, heart or liver recipients often face more limited options for life extension. Nevertheless, even the rates of nonadherence among heart and liver recipients, which stand at 15 to 20 cases per 100 PPY and 8 cases per 100 PPY respectively, could raise clinical concerns. These rates

Transplant recipient type	Non-adherence rate	Impact	Significance
Kidney	38	Fewer demanding psychosocial standards and graft loss effects	High percentage of nonadherence which could affect graft survival.
Heart	15–20	Psychosocial requirements, effects of graft loss	Despite minimal nonadherence rates patient results are nevertheless affected.
Liver	8	High psychosocial standards and serious graft loss effects	High rates of nonadherence, which impact graft survival.
Tobacco Use	5–6	Impactful but relatively lower	Use of tobacco increases posttransplant morbidity and mortality.

Table 1.
Comparative rates of immunosuppressant nonadherence across different transplant recipient types.

are potentially deemed unacceptable. Notably, all these rates surpass the incidence of tobacco use, a potent contributor to post transplant morbidity and mortality. Even at its comparatively lower level of 5 to 6 patients per 100 PPY, tobacco use still significantly impacts patient outcomes after transplantation. **Table 1** depicts about the type of transplant recipient, rate, impact and its significance.

5. Strategies to improve organ transplantation

The research examines a multifaceted exploration of key approaches aimed at elevating the success and effectiveness of organ transplantation procedures [22]. This critical discourse underscores the paramount importance of optimizing various facets of the transplantation process to enhance patient outcomes and the longevity of graft survival. The monarchy of immunosuppression management, show a vital role in suppressing the recipient's immune response to prevent graft rejection. Advancements in personalized immunosuppressive regimens, often combining multiple medications with distinct mechanisms of action, strive to strike a delicate balance between minimizing the risk of rejection and avoiding over-immunosuppression-related complications. Additionally, targeted therapies that focus on specific immune pathways hold promise in mitigating the adverse effects of immunosuppression while maintaining graft tolerance. Moreover, the research navigates the advanced tissue typing and cross matching techniques enable a more nuanced evaluation of compatibility between donor and recipient, reducing the risk of immune-mediated graft rejection. Thus this encapsulates a holistic perspective on the dynamic approaches that converge to create a transformative impact on the success of organ transplantation. By synergizing innovations in immunosuppression, organ preservation, and compatibility optimization, this section underscores the unyielding commitment of the medical community to elevate transplantation outcomes, ultimately enhancing the quality of life for recipients and advancing the frontiers of transplantation medicine.

5.1 Advancements in immunosuppressive drugs

Advancements in immunosuppressive drugs have played a pivotal role in mitigating immune reactions against non-ABO antigens in the perspective of organ transplantation [23]. These drugs are designed to moderate the recipient's immune response, thus dropping the hazard of graft rejection and improving the long-term existence of transplanted organs. One key category of immunosuppressive drugs includes calcineurin inhibitors such as cyclosporine and tacrolimus. These drugs work by inhibiting the activity of calcineurin, a crucial enzyme in T cell activation. By dampening T cell responses, these drugs help prevent the immune system from recognizing the transplanted organ as foreign. This mechanism is particularly relevant in reducing immune reactions against non-ABO antigens, as T cells are major contributors to immune-mediated graft rejection. Another class of immunosuppressants comprises mTOR inhibitors like sirolimus and everolimus. These drugs target the mammalian target of rapamycin (mTOR) path, which normalizes cell proliferation and immune responses. By inhibiting mTOR, these drugs impede T cell activation and proliferation, further reducing the immune system's ability to mount a strong response against non-ABO antigens. Moreover, Corticosteroids like prednisone, have been used for decades as immunosuppressive agents. They exert broad anti-inflammatory effects and can suppress various components of the immune response, including T cell activity and antibody production. While their use is related with a range of side effects, comprising metabolic disturbances and increased infection risk, corticosteroids remain an essential tool in managing immune reactions after transplantation.

Consequently, the emergence of targeted biologic agents has ushered in a new era of immunosuppression. Moreover, monoclonal antibodies like basiliximab and alemtuzumab specifically target certain immune cell surface markers, effectively depleting or suppressing the activity of these cells. These agents offer a more precise means of immune suppression, allowing for better control over immune reactions against non-ABO antigens. Thus, advancements in immunosuppressive drugs have enabled clinicians to tailor treatment regimens to individual patient needs, optimizing the balance between immune suppression and the risk of infections or other complications. By specifically targeting pathways involved in immune responses, these drugs help minimize the risk of immune reactions against non-ABO antigens, thus enhancing graft survival and improving the overall success of organ transplantation [24]. However, the challenge lies in maintaining a delicate equilibrium between suppressing the immune response and ensuring the recipient's ability to fight infections and other challenges. Ongoing research continues to refine immunosuppressive strategies and develop novel agents to further enhance transplantation outcomes.

The allocation of scarce donor organs is a deeply challenging and ethically charged endeavor, as it involves balancing equitable access to life-saving treatments with the imperative to maximize positive outcomes for recipients. Blood group compatibility, particularly in ABO and RhD systems, is a fundamental criterion in organ allocation, aimed at minimizing the risk of graft rejection and improving transplantation success rates. However, this approach raises ethical dilemmas, as prioritizing recipients with compatible blood groups can inadvertently disadvantage those with less common or rare blood types. This can result in longer wait times for some patients and potentially compromise their health and quality of life. One ethical concern pertains to fairness and distributive justice. Allocating organs primarily based on blood group compatibility might disproportionately benefit individuals with more prevalent blood types, leaving those with rarer blood types at a disadvantage. This challenge is especially relevant when considering the global diversity of blood groups and the varying prevalence of different types within different populations.

Additionally, the ethical discourse extends to the consideration of medical urgency and the principle of utility. Balancing medical urgency against blood group compatibility raises questions about the ethical imperative to save lives versus the importance of minimizing post-transplant complications. Furthermore, the ethical complexities intersect with the broader context of organ trafficking, commercialization, and illegal organ trade. As the ultimatum for organs exceeds the obtainable source, there is a risk that the focus on blood group compatibility could exacerbate the incentive for illegal organ transactions and exploitation, compromising the ethical foundations of organ allocation.

These ethical challenges should navigate transplant societies, ethicists, and policymakers must carefully deliberate on allocation criteria that balance compatibility, medical need, fairness, and justice. It is imperative to uphold transparency in organ allocation processes, engage in public discourse, and consider innovative approaches that ensure equitable access to transplantation for all individuals, regardless of their blood group compatibility. Ultimately, addressing these ethical concerns requires a delicate balance between optimizing transplantation outcomes and upholding principles of justice, autonomy, and human dignity in the allocation of life-saving organs.

Moreover, transplantation techniques and strategies evolve to enhance compatibility and minimize graft rejection, the broader societal landscape experiences various positive transformations. Improved transplantation outcomes contribute to a significant improvement in the overall quality of life for transplant recipients. As graft rejection rates decrease due to enhanced compatibility measures, recipients experience longer graft survival, reduced need for re-transplantation, and decreased rates of post-transplant complications. This leads to improved physical health, reduced dependency on medical interventions, and a greater ability to engage in daily activities, work, and social interactions. Transplant recipients often regain a sense of normalcy and the ability to actively participate in society, contributing to a higher quality of life and increased overall well-being. On a societal level, the positive impact extends to healthcare systems and resource allocation. Successful transplantation outcomes reduce the burden on healthcare resources by decreasing the need for prolonged hospital stays, ongoing medical interventions, and expensive treatments associated with graft failure or complications. This optimization of healthcare utilization frees up resources that can be redirected toward other medical needs, ultimately enhancing the efficiency and sustainability of healthcare systems. Furthermore, improved transplantation outcomes have a positive ripple effect on the workforce and economy. Successful transplant recipients who return to work and productive activities contribute to a more robust labor force and increased economic productivity. This, in turn, generates a positive economic impact over augmented tax profits, condensed dependence on social welfare platforms, and improved economic growth. Beyond the immediate health and economic benefits, the societal impact extends to public perception and awareness of transplantation. Positive outcomes and reduced graft rejection rates reinforce public confidence in transplantation as a viable and life-transforming medical solution. This may lead to increased organ donation rates, as the public witnesses the tangible benefits of their organ donations in the form of successful transplant stories.

Moreover, the societal impact of improved transplantation outcomes and reduced graft rejection rates is multifaceted and profound. From individual recipients experiencing a better quality of life to healthcare systems benefiting from optimized resource allocation, and from an enhanced labor force to heightened public trust in transplantation, these advancements catalyze a positive cycle of improved well-being and societal well-being. As research and innovation continue, the potential for even greater societal benefits through transplantation remains a promising avenue for medical progress and societal advancement.

The focus must be directed toward deciphering the underlying mechanisms that intricately influence the acceptance or rejection of grafts by unveiling the immunological significance of blood types. Through an exploration of the complex interplay between antibodies, antigens, and the immune response, the chapter underscores how even subtle variations in blood type antigens can incite profound immunological reactions, ultimately shaping the success of transplantation outcomes. The clinical implications of blood group matching in the context of organ transplantation are underscored, as this investigation sheds light on the profound influence of blood compatibility on graft survival. In addition, the discourse extends to the horizon of emerging advancements in immunogenetics and immunosuppressive therapies, offering a promising arsenal to surmount the challenges posed by blood group disparities. In sum, this chapter constitutes an invaluable resource for healthcare practitioners and researchers, providing strategic insights that can propel the refinement of matching strategies and elevate the overall efficacy of transplantation practices in the dynamic landscape of medical science.

The recognition of non-ABO antigens, from the Rh and other blood group systems, poses a potential risk for immune responses during blood transfusions and organ transplantation. These immune reactions can result in hemolysis, transfusion reactions, and other adverse effects that compromise patient safety. While ABO compatibility remains a fundamental consideration, addressing non-ABO antigens, especially within the HLA system, holds equal significance in ensuring the success of these medical interventions. The importance of minimizing immune responses against these antigens cannot be overstated, as it directly influences the compatibility and acceptance of transplanted organs. Furthermore, this principle extends to treatments involving bone marrow and stem cell transplantation, where preventing immune reactions against non-ABO antigens is pivotal in preventing harmful graft-versus-host responses. By meticulously addressing and managing non-ABO antigen compatibility, healthcare professionals strive to enhance patient outcomes, reduce complications, and optimize the effectiveness of transfusions and transplantation therapies. Further study in this area has the possibility to enhance patient satisfaction, reduce graft rejection rates, and enhance transplantation procedures. Researchers may contribute to the creation of novel medicines, individualized methods, and a greater comprehension of the immune system's function in transplantation by unraveling the complex immunological connections caused by blood group antigens.

Author details

B. Pushpa[1*], R.A. Shanmugha Priya[2], Ushus S. Kumar[1] and J. Saminathan[1]

1 Department of Biomedical Engineering, SRM Institute of Science and Technology, Chennai, India

2 Transfusion Medicine, Kauvery Hospital, Chennai, India

*Address all correspondence to: pushpaazhagesan@gmail.com

References

[1] Amoroso A et al. HLA and AB0 polymorphisms may influence SARS-CoV-2 infection and COVID-19 severity. Transplantation. 2021;**105**(1):193-200

[2] Gotlieb N et al. The promise of machine learning applications in solid organ transplantation. NPJ Digital Medicine. 2022;**5**(1):89. DOI: 10.1038/s41746-022-00637-2

[3] McCormack D. The times and spaces of transplantation: Queercrip histories as futurities. Medical Humanities. 2021;**47**(4):397-406

[4] Angelico R, Trapani S, Manzia TM, Lombardini L, Tisone G, Cardillo M. The COVID-19 outbreak in Italy: Initial implications for organ transplantation programs. American Journal of Transplantation. 2020;**20**(7):1780-1784. DOI: 10.1111/ajt.15904

[5] Jain S, Ahlstrom D. Technology legitimacy and the legitimacy of technology: The case of chronic kidney disease therapies. Journal of Engineering and Technology Management. 2021;**62**:101653. DOI: 10.1016/j.jengtecman.2021.101653

[6] Pendu JL, Breiman A, Rocher J, Dion M, Ruvoën-Clouet N. ABO blood types and COVID-19: Spurious, anecdotal, or truly important relationships? A reasoned review of available data. Viruses. 2021;**13**(2):160

[7] Ukirde V, Usulumarty D, Maru H, Billa V. Are weak blood groups important to look for in kidney transplantation? A case report on interchanging blood groups. Indian Journal of Transplantation. 2020;**14**(4):355. DOI: 10.4103/ijot.ijot_92_20

[8] Callemeyn J, Lamarthée B, Koenig A, Koshy P, Thaunat O, Naesens M. Allorecognition and the spectrum of kidney transplant rejection. Kidney International. 2022;**101**(4):692-710. DOI: 10.1016/j.kint.2021.11.029

[9] Gao H, Misevic G, LIBO J, Medicine Biotechnology Co., Ltd. Jiangyin, Jiangsu 214400, China. Microchip technology applications for blood group analysis. Blood and Genomics. 2020;**4**(2):83-95. DOI: 10.46701/BG.2020022020109

[10] Kucirka LM, Lauer SA, Laeyendecker O, Boon D, Lessler J. Variation in false-negative rate of reverse transcriptase polymerase chain reaction–based SARS-CoV-2 tests by time since exposure. Annals of Internal Medicine. 2020;**173**(4):262-267

[11] Opara ER. Review on knowledge of issues of rhesus incompatibility among nigerians. Opera. 2023;**3**(2)

[12] Altayar M et al. Prevalence and association of transfusion transmitted infections with ABO and Rh blood groups among blood donors in the Western region of Saudi Arabia: A 7-year retrospective analysis. Medicina. 2022;**58**(7):857. DOI: 10.3390/medicina58070857

[13] Arnaiz-Villena A et al. Evolution and molecular interactions of major histocompatibility complex (MHC)-G, −E and -F genes. Cellular and Molecular Life Sciences. 2022;**79**(8):464. DOI: 10.1007/s00018-022-04491-z

[14] Tersigni C et al. Role of human leukocyte antigens at the feto-maternal interface in normal and pathological pregnancy: An update. International

Journal of Molecular Sciences. 2020;**21**(13):4756. DOI: 10.3390/ijms21134756

[15] Robinson RA, McMurran C, McCully ML, Cole DK. Engineering soluble T-cell receptors for therapy. The FEBS Journal. 2021;**288**(21):6159-6173. DOI: 10.1111/febs.15780

[16] Accolla RS, Ramia E, Tedeschi A, Forlani G. CIITA-driven MHC class II expressing tumor cells as antigen presenting cell performers: Toward the construction of an optimal anti-tumor vaccine. Frontiers in Immunology. 2019;**10**:1806. DOI: 10.3389/fimmu.2019.01806

[17] Lemieux W, Mohammadhassanzadeh H, Klement W, Daniel C, Sapir-Pichhadze R. Matchmaker, matchmaker make me a match: Opportunities and challenges in optimizing compatibility of HLA eplets in transplantation. International Journal of Immunogenetics. 2021;**48**(2):135-144. DOI: 10.1111/iji.12525

[18] Stowell CP, Stowell SR. Biologic roles of the ABH and Lewis histo-blood group antigens part I: Infection and immunity. Vox Sanguinis. 2019;**114**(5):426-442. DOI: 10.1111/vox.12787

[19] Kummer L et al. Vascular Signaling in allogenic solid organ transplantation – The role of endothelial cells. Frontiers in Physiology. 2020;**11**:443. DOI: 10.3389/fphys.2020.00443

[20] Santarsiero D, Aiello S. The complement system in kidney transplantation. Cell. 2023;**12**(5):791

[21] Kostalova B, Mala-Ladova K, Sulkova SD, Denhaerynck K, De Geest S, Maly J. Comparison of different methods to assess tacrolimus concentration intra-patient variability as potential marker of medication non-adherence. Frontiers in Pharmacology. 2022;**13**:973564. DOI: 10.3389/fphar.2022.973564

[22] Beheshtizadeh N et al. Vascular endothelial growth factor (VEGF) delivery approaches in regenerative medicine. Biomedicine & Pharmacotherapy. 2023;**166**:115301. DOI: 10.1016/j.biopha.2023.115301

[23] Hong H, Duque MA, Mana AFA, Wu Y. Noninfectious transfusion-associated adverse events. Annals of Blood. 2022;7:19-19. DOI: 10.21037/aob-21-83

[24] Cheng C-H et al. ABO-incompatible liver transplantation: State of art and future perspectives. Current Pharmaceutical Design. 2020;**26**(28):3406-3417. DOI: 10.2174/1381612826666200506094539

Chapter 7

Mitochondrial Dysfunction-Triggered Innate Immune Response and Its Therapeutic Implications

Yinghong He, Boyuan Shen and Xiang Zhou

Abstract

Mitochondria are essential organelles that play a pivotal role in a variety of biological processes, including energy production, metabolism, cell death, and inflammation. Interestingly, within these organelles lies a hidden component with the potential to activate the innate immune system: mitochondrial DNA (mtDNA). Pathogenic microorganisms invasion or danger signals can cause mitochondrial structures to become abnormal or dysfunctional, leading to the release of mtDNA into the cytoplasm, which in turn triggers the innate immune response. The leakage of mtDNA into the cytoplasm activates the cGAS-STING signaling pathway, which results in the production of type I interferons and inflammatory cytokines. Additionally, when mtDNA is oxidized, it can activate the NLRP3 inflammasome, leading to the initiation of various cell death mechanisms, such as pyroptosis. In this review, we delve into the role of mtDNA released from dysfunctional mitochondria as a potent activator of the immune system, which can lead to a cascade of inflammatory reactions. The engagement of the STING and NLRP3 inflammasomes is intricately linked to the development of inflammation, autoimmune disorders, and cancer. Targeting these pathways with specific agonists or inhibitors holds promise as a therapeutic strategy for a range of immune-related diseases and cancer.

Keywords: innate immunity, mitochondrial dysfunction, mtDNA, STING, NLRP3, pyroptosis, autoimmune disease, inflammatory disease, cancer

1. Introduction

Mitochondria are important organelles that are ubiquitously present in eukaryotic cells and have a unique double-membrane structure, participating in various physiological processes such as cell metabolism, signal transduction, and apoptosis [1]. One specific genome of mitochondria, mtDNA, encodes essential protein subunits of the oxidative phosphorylation system, including the electron transport chain (ETC; complexes I-IV) and ATP synthase (complex V). Its main function is to carry out aerobic respiration, oxidize, and decompose the organic matter in the cells under the action

IntechOpen

of enzymes to release energy and produce adenosine triphosphate (ATP) required for the life activities of the cells [2]. When mutations occur in mtDNA and the nuclear genome (nDNA), which jointly control the function of mitochondria, mitochondrial dysfunction may be caused [3]. So far, mitochondria have been proved to play an important role in innate immunity. For example, they promote immune cell activation and antimicrobial defense by regulating signal transduction and effector functions and trigger inflammatory responses when cells and tissues are damaged [4, 5].

The cGAS-STING, as an important innate immune pathway in cells, is closely related to mtDNA. When cells are invaded by microorganisms or receive danger signals, mitochondrial structure and function become abnormal, releasing mtDNA. mtDNA is recognized and bound by cGAS in the cytoplasm, activating the STING pathway to initiate the transcription and expression of related genes such as type I interferon (IFN), thereby activating the immune response [6]. The excessive activation of the NLRP3 inflammasome is closely related to the occurrence of various inflammatory diseases and autoimmune diseases. Studies have shown that oxidized mtDNA can bind to NLRP3 and activate the NLRP3 inflammasome [7]. This review will concentrate on the mechanism of mtDNA as a stimulus of the immune system to activate the cGAS-STING pathway and inflammasomes and reveals how mtDNA is exposed in the cytoplasm. Numerous evidence indicates that inflammation-associated illnesses are primarily centered around mtDNA. We intend to clarify the targets of diseases related to mtDNA and explore new treatment possibilities that are based on various studies.

2. mtDNA as a stimulus of the immune system

Mitochondria, as common organelles, are generally manifested as short rod-shaped or spherical granules of varying sizes and have a double-membrane structure. Its outer membrane distinguishes the mitochondrial matrix from the cytoplasm, and the inner membrane folds inward to form cristae, which is the main site of biochemical reactions within mitochondria. The inner mitochondrial membrane encloses the mitochondrial matrix, which contains not only many proteins such as enzymes required for mitochondrial biochemical reactions but also the mitochondrial own genetic material and genetic system, namely mitochondrial DNA, RNA, and ribosomes [8]. It is precisely because of its unique genetic system distinct from other organelles that the origin of mitochondria has been widely discussed, among which the endosymbiotic theory occupies a major position [9].

Since 2004, Collins et al. [10] found that injecting mtDNA into the joints of mice will trigger local inflammation, while injecting nuclear DNA does not elicit this response. In addition, they detected the presence of extracellular mtDNA in the synovial fluid of patients with rheumatoid arthritis, but no such phenomenon occurred in the normal control group. This discovery has led to further studies of mtDNA in the field related to immunology. And more and more evidence indicates that the leakage behavior of mitochondrial DNA after damage is one of the main driving factors of inflammation, and more investigations and studies clearly indicate that it is related to more and more inflammatory diseases by stimulating innate immune pathways.

Intracellular nucleic acid sensors play an indispensable role in innate immunity. Current studies have shown that mtDNA mainly stimulates innate immunity through the following three pathways: the TLR9 sensing pathway, the NLRP3 binding oxidized mtDNA pathway, and the cGAS-STING pathway. TLR9 has been proven to be a PRR that can specifically recognize CpG fragments present in mtDNA and can trigger the upregulation of NF-κB through this pathway [11–14]. The NLRP3 inflammasome can also recognize mtDNA. When mitochondria have dysfunction and are released into the cytoplasm, it can directly stimulate the activation of NLRP3 inflammasome, promote the secretion of IL-1β/IL-18, and lead to pyroptosis of cells [15–18]. At the same time, the cGAS-STING pathway can also capture mtDNA leaked into the cytoplasm. The activation of this pathway can trigger the release of type I interferons and a series of inflammatory responses [19, 20]. This pathway will be further discussed in this review.

However, the release of mtDNA is a prerequisite for initiating innate immunity, as the membrane structure of mitochondria isolates mtDNA from the cytoplasm. Although the factors that determine the mode of mtDNA release and the effective contents of mitochondrial release are still unclear at present, its release mechanism has gradually been revealed in recent studies. The predominant observation of mtDNA release is currently attributed to the formation of large pores by the proteins BAX and BAK during the process of mitochondrial-mediated apoptosis [21, 22]. A recent study on BAX/BAK found that the mutual regulation of BAX and BAK is involved in the regulation of the rate of pore formation on the membrane during cell transfer, further leading to the release of mitochondrial DNA [23]. Although the specific mechanism of BAX/BAK initiating the apoptotic cascade reaction has not been clarified, it clearly demonstrates the decisive role that BAX and BAK play in the apoptotic process.

The voltage-dependent anion channel (VDAC) in the mitochondrial permeability transition pore (mPTP) has also been observed to play a role in mitochondrial release [24]. In early studies, the formation of pores by VDAC1 and VDAC3 or their oligomers was considered to be related to the release of mtDNA. This pathway activates VDAC protein oligomerization through mPTP and binds to oxidized mtDNA, and releases it from mitochondria to activate NLRP3. However, recent studies have shown that VDAC2 also plays a regulatory role in promoting mitochondrial release [25]. However, the influencing factors that initiate the VDAC release of mtDNA pathway are not clear. In some studies, it is proposed that it is not regulated by a single factor, which also implies that this pathway may be regulated by more extensive factors, and perhaps this release pathway plays an important role in cellular immunity.

In any case, due to the environment prone to oxidative damage caused by its proximity to the electron transport chain [26, 27], the unique structure or errors caused during the processes such as replication, copying, and repair, as well as various possible mitochondrial autophagy defects, autophagosome/lysosome defects, etc., all provide sufficient conditions for the recognition of intracellular nucleic acid sensors and the release of downstream interferons. Although studies on the release of mtDNA in recent years have mentioned the mechanisms of mitochondrial release channel formation that may play a major role, they are still limited, and the more extensive and comprehensive influencing factors and initiation mechanisms of mtDNA release will need to be further explored.

3. Activation of the cGAS-STING signal depends on mtDNA

The recognition of exogenous DNA is one of the key factors for the activation of innate immunity. The specific binding of multiple pattern recognition receptors (PRRs) to various pathogen-associated molecular patterns (PAMPs) triggers the activation of downstream cascade pathways. These pathogen-associated molecules often come from foreign substances recognized by cells such as bacteria and viruses. PRRs include a variety of PAMPs sensing proteins, including toll-like receptors (TLRs), inflammasomes, RNA sensors of the RIG-I-like receptor (RLR) family, and DNA sensors such as cyclic GMP-AMP synthase (cGAS). Among them, the signaling pathway formed by cyclic cGAS and stimulator of interferon genes (STING) plays an important role in mammals [28].

cGAS is a member of the evolutionarily ancient cGAS/dncv-like nucleotide transferase (CD-NTase) family. Proteins of this family can synthesize various cyclic oligonucleotide second messengers in response to pathogen invasion. (cGAS–STING Signaling) cGAS in mammals structurally contains a nucleotide transferase domain, which can bind to the sugar-phosphate backbone of dsDNA, thereby inducing the formation of cGAS dimers [29]. After the formation of the 2:2 cGAS-DNA complex, it catalyzes the synthesis of cyclic GMP-AMP (cGAMP) from guanosine triphosphate (GTP) and ATP. STING is an endoplasmic reticulum membrane protein containing four transmembrane domains. Under normal conditions, it exists in the form of a tight dimer linked by two STING molecules. The dimer contains a binding domain for cGAMP. After the STING dimer binds to cGAMP, the structure is rearranged to facilitate the oligomerization of STING on the endoplasmic reticulum membrane. The disulfide bridge across the STING dimer and the palmitoylation of cysteine residues C88 and C91 further promote oligomerization. Subsequently, STING is transported to the Golgi apparatus through the Golgi intermediate compartment and recruits TANK-binding kinase 1 (TBK1) through the highly conserved TBK1-binding PxPLR motif at the carboxyl-terminal tail of STING on the Golgi apparatus. After phosphorylation of TBK1, it in turn activates the phosphorylation of the adjacent pLxIS motif (where p represents a hydrophilic residue) on STING, allowing it to recruit interferon regulatory factor 3 (IRF3) and phosphorylate it through TBK1. The phosphorylated IRF3 then dimerizes and translocates to the nucleus to activate the expression of type I interferons and downstream interferon-stimulated genes.

We find that the dsDNA binding ability of cGAS is the key to the initiation of the entire signaling pathway. It is not difficult for us to think that mtDNA, as dsDNA, also has the ability to activate the cGAS-STING pathway. This is exactly the case. cGAS has not only been proven to be activated by viral DNA in many studies on antiviral research, but also has been proven to be activated by mtDNA in many studies in recent years. In 2015, White et al. [30] found in the study of cell death that the deficiency of mitochondrial transcription factor A (TFAM) promoted the release of mtDNA from mitochondria into the cytoplasm, which activated cGAS and triggered the type I interferon response. Similarly, in a study provided by Hu et al. [31] in 2023 on the ATM gene and immune checkpoint blockade therapy, it was also found that the cGAS-STING pathway was activated due to mtDNA. The knockout of the ATM gene in this study significantly upregulated the expression of ISGs (interferon-stimulated genes) and confirmed that a large amount of DNA present in the cytoplasm came from mitochondria. In further studies, they discovered the downregulation of TFAM and believed that it played an important role in the ATM inhibition-induced mitochondrial DNA release and activation of the cGAS-STING pathway. Herpes simplex virus-1 (HSV-1) and vesicular stomatitis virus (VSV) infections can not only directly trigger the type I interferon response as pathogens, but also cause mtDNA stress and TFAM depletion, which also causes mtDNA to leak into the cytoplasm and be recognized by cGAS, triggering the cGAS-STING signal [32, 33]. In several studies on Mycobacterium tuberculosis infection, researchers discovered that mitochondrial stress and the release of mtDNA in addition to mycobacterial DNA triggered cGAS activation and subsequent type I interferon responses [34–37]. Brokatzky et al. [37] also provided a report on pathogen-induced mitochondrial permeability. In this study, they found that various pathogens can induce the release of mtDNA. Although the release mechanism is still unclear at present, they detected the activation of the effective cGAS-STING pathway and the secretion of downstream cytokines. In addition, in the study by Aarreberg et al. [38], it was found that IL-1b released by cells with activated inflammatory pathways induces the release of mtDNA in surrounding cells, activating their cGAS-STING-dependent type I interferon response. This study emphasized for the first time the key role of mtDNA release in cross-cell communication.

mtDNA is released under pathological conditions such as oxidative stress, genotoxic stress, high levels of pro-inflammatory factors, viral infection, and mitochondrial dysfunction and subsequently activates the cGAS-STING pathway. Although most studies on the cGAS-STING pathway triggered by mtDNA leakage have not yet been able to resolve the mechanism of mtDNA release, the clear phenomena of mtDNA leakage and cGAS-STING pathway activation have often been observed and further confirmed in control experiments. These studies undoubtedly reveal the important role of mtDNA in the activation of innate immune pathways and provide a powerful reference for subsequent studies on inflammation.

4. Therapies targeting mtDNA-dependent cGAS-STING activity

Interest in mtDNA within the realms of inflammation and immunity research is growing steadily, offering novel perspectives for the management of associated conditions. As mentioned earlier, the specific release mechanism of mtDNA in various pathological manifestations is not yet clear; however, in recent years, the cGAS-STING signaling pathway has gradually become clear. The type I interferon response triggered by this pathway can not only promote the anti-infection ability by enhancing the function of T cells, but also act on the tumor microenvironment, recruit, and activate immune cells to function. Therefore, the cGAS-STING signaling pathway plays a key role in the body's anti-infection, tumor immunity, autoimmune diseases, and aging-related inflammation. Also for this reason, the research and development of inhibitors and agonists targeting this pathway can achieve immunotherapy for related diseases caused by the cGAS-STING pathway by promoting and blocking the signal transduction of a certain link in this signaling pathway (**Figure 1**).

Many reports have pointed out that existing metal ions such as manganese and zinc can act as agonists of the cGAS pathway and have shown good agonistic effects in experiments. However, because the required concentration is prone to pose a safety threat to the human body, there are no relevant reports on such cGAS agonists being studied as drugs [39]. The cGAS regulatory factor, GTPase-activating protein SH3 domain-binding protein 1, has been proved to promote the formation of the cGAS-DNA complex. Liu et al. [40] discovered an inhibitor EGCG that can inhibit G3BP1. This inhibitor can inhibit the recognition and binding of cGAS to dsDNA, thereby inhibiting the release of downstream type I interferons and the activation of related ISGs. Currently, this inhibitor has been proved to have an effective inhibitory effect in animal models of autoimmune diseases and Aicardi-Goutières syndrome. It is also found that aspirin has the effect of inhibiting the autoimmune response in AGS patient cells and mouse models [41]. Aspirin can inhibit the enzymatic activity of

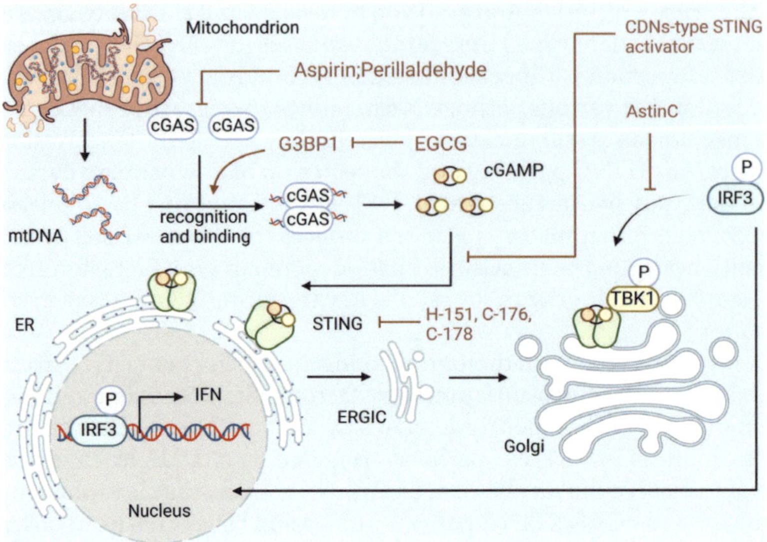

Figure 1.
mtDNA-dependent activation of the cGAS-STING pathway and drug targets. After mtDNA leakage from mitochondria due to cellular intrinsic or extrinsic factors, cGAS as a DNA receptor will recognize mtDNA and form cGAS-DNA complexes and catalyze the synthesis of cGAMP. STING on the ER receives the signal from cGAMP and is transported to Golgi via ERGIC to bind to TBK1 and phosphorylate it, followed by the recruitment of IRF3, which is phosphorylated using TBK1. IRF3 is activated and then enters the nucleus of the cell to activate the downstream type I interferon response. Among them, inhibitors such as aspirin and perillaldehyde can inhibit cGAS enzyme activity, EGCG can indirectly inhibit the recognition binding process between cGAS and dsDNA by inhibiting G3BP1, drugs such as H-151, C-176, C-177 can inhibit STING molecular palmitoylation, CDNs-type STING activator can activate STING by binding to STING, and drugs such as AstinC block the recruitment of IRF3.

cGAS by promoting the acetylation of lysine residues (Lys384, Lys394, and Lys414) at positions 384, 394, and 414 of cGAS, thereby inhibiting the activation of downstream signaling pathways. Perillaldehyde is a natural monoterpene compound extracted from perilla. Chu et al. [42] reported that perillaldehyde inhibits innate immunity caused by DNA in the cytoplasm by inhibiting cGAS activity. In this report, perillaldehyde promoted the infection effect of HSV-1 on mice, and the down-regulation of ISG expressions such as Cxcl10, Isg15, and IFIT3 promoted by perillaldehyde was found in the mouse model of AGS disease.

STING, as an important regulatory protein in this signaling pathway, its transport mechanism, and binding mechanism are both important targets for inhibitors and agonists targeting this pathway. Currently, for the STING binding region, researchers have developed AstinC from aster to block the process of STING recruiting IRF3 [43]. This compound can inhibit the recruitment and activation of IRF3 by competitively binding to the STING CTD region, thereby inhibiting downstream pathway changes, and significant relief of spontaneous inflammation has been observed in the Trex1$^{-/-}$ mouse model. And for the palmitoylation of the cysteine residue of STING, researchers have screened out compounds such as H-151, C-176, and C-178 to prevent the palmitoylation of the STING molecule [44], thereby inhibiting downstream signal changes such as TBK1 phosphorylation and significantly improving the progression of autoimmune diseases in mouse models. Promoting STING translocation and activating STING to exert a signaling effect play a key immunotherapeutic role in anti-pathogen infection and cancer treatment. ADU-S100, as the first CDNs-type STING activator to enter clinical trials, has a stronger interferon response agonistic effect than natural CDNs. However, its clinical trial has now been terminated due to its poor anti-tumor performance. Still, other CDNs analogues are gradually being developed, and most have shown good anti-tumor ability in the early stage of research. For example, the newly developed MK-1454 by Merck has shown excellent safety and therapeutic effects in combination with pembrolizumab in patients with advanced solid tumors and lymphomas and has entered phase II clinical trials. 3′,3′-cyclicAMP, as a novel agonist of STING, also shows good therapeutic effects on hepatocellular carcinoma, achieving the promotion of tumor regression and increased apoptosis of tumor cells [45].

Additionally, the important molecules and release mechanisms that mtDNA release may rely on have gradually emerged, enabling the research on disease treatment targeting the mtDNA-dependent cGAS-STING pathway to be carried out. Moreover, the proposal of this pathway seems to have a greater impact than we imagined. Systemic lupus erythematosus (SLE) is a typical autoimmune disease mainly caused by abnormal activation of the immune system. The specific cause of this disease is not yet clear, but new evidence indicates that the level of mtDNA in the serum of SLE patients is ten times higher than that of normal people, and abnormal accumulation of SNPs in SLE patients has been detected, which is likely due to the imbalance of mitochondrial homeostasis [46, 47]. Furthermore, some studies have shown that elevated levels of cGAMP were detected in some SLE patients, but this phenomenon was not detected in rheumatoid arthritis patients and healthy controls [48], and cGAS was also identified as the main factor for IFN expression in SLE in another report. This report [49] discovered and proved that the absence of the hypoxia-inducible factor (HIF)-mediated mitophagy pathway led to the accumulation of erythrocytes carrying mitochondria in SLE patients. This phenomenon activated the cGAS pathway in macrophages and the subsequent type I interferon response, causing the typical pathological manifestations in SLE patients. All these evidences emphasize that the release of mtDNA with the activation of the cGAS-STNG pathway may play an important role in the pathogenic mechanism of SLE [50, 51].

Immune checkpoint blockade therapy has made significant progress in the current field of cancer immunotherapy. Abnormal cell metabolism plays a crucial role in the regulation of the immune response of cancer cells. The enhanced lipid synthesis ability meets the needs of rapid growth and tumorigenesis of cancer cells. Adenosine 50 -triphosphate citrate lyase (ACLY), as one of the key enzymes for de novo fatty acid synthesis, has been studied in the report by Xiang et al. [52]. In this study, they proposed that the inhibition of ACLY led to the accumulation of PUFAs in cancer cells, further promoting lipid peroxidation and peroxidation and damage leakage of mitochondrial DNA. The peroxidation and release of mtDNA upregulated the expression of PD-L1 by activating the cGAS-STING signal, thereby mediating the immune escape of cancer cells. However, the cGAS-STING pathway plays a dual role in tumor immune regulation. Although it can promote the killing of T cells through the interferon response, at the same time, as shown in this study, it can promote the immune escape of cancer cells. Therefore, immunotherapy targeting this pathway needs to be combined with other treatment regimens, and perhaps good results will be expected.

Through the research on the cGAS-STING pathway stimulated by targeting mtDNA, the therapeutic effect of radiotherapy on cancer has been newly improved in the study by Li et al. In a report [24] they provided in 2023, TRIM21 promotes VDAC2 degradation by increasing its k48-linked ubiquitination. The reduction of VDAC2 inhibits the release of mtDNA, thereby indirectly regulating the type I interferon immune response generated by the cGAS-STING pathway. This study specifically located the regulatory effect of TRIM21 on the cGAS-STING pathway during radiation to the inhibition of mtDNA release and proposed the possibility of enhancing the tumor immune response through drugs targeting TRIM21.

In conclusion, these research progresses are providing valuable data and the theoretical basis for the immunotherapy regimens targeting the mtDNA-mediated cGAS-STING pathway and providing broader perspectives and ideas for more immune-related disease treatment methods.

5. Oxidized mtDNA as an activator of the NLRP3 inflammasome

The activation of the NLRP3 inflammasome is a complex and strictly regulated process involving two crucial signals: the priming signal and the activation signal [53]. In the priming signal, it is typically induced by microbial components, cytokines (such as tumor necrosis factor-α), etc. Through specific PRRs like TLRs, NLRs, and cytokine receptors, they recognize PAMPs and DAMPs, leading to the activation of the NF-κB signaling pathway and the upregulation of NLRP3, Pro-IL-1β, and Pro-IL-18. In the activation signal, it induces the assembly and activation of the NLRP3 inflammasome [54, 55]. When cells are stimulated by the internal and external environment, it results in mitochondrial dysfunction, oxidative damage to mtDNA, and its release into the cytoplasm. Oxidized mtDNA can bind to NLRP3, causing conformational changes in NLRP3 and its interaction with the adaptor protein ASC and the effector protein pro-caspase-1 to form an inflammasome complex. The activated caspase-1 can cleave pro-IL-1β and pro-IL-18 into active IL-1β and IL-18 and release them outside the cell, triggering an inflammatory response [56]. Activated caspase-1 also cleaves gasdermin D (GSDMD), thereby triggering a specific form of cell death, pyroptosis [57].

In 2011, Nakahira et al. [58] reported that in mouse bone marrow-derived macrophages, the depletion of beclin 1 and LC3B led to the accumulation of dysfunctional persistent mitochondria, showing excessive ROS. Under the stimulation of lipopolysaccharide (LPS) or ATP, these mitochondria released mtDNA into the cytoplasm. Nakahira et al. also suggested that NLRP3 functions both in the middle and downstream of mtDNA release and can facilitate the formation of mPTP on mitochondria, thereby releasing mtDNA. In 2012, Shimada et al. [7] reported that during macrophage apoptosis, mtDNA was released and bound to NLRP3. And in the process of mtDNA binding to NLRP3, NLRP3 has a greater propensity to bind oxidized mtDNA. These two reports concluded that mitochondrial dysfunction releases mtDNA and generates excessive ROS, along with the binding of oxidized mtDNA to NLRP3. According to the research of Xian et al. [59]. In 2022, when mtDNA is oxidized to form Ox-mtDNA, Ox-mtDNA binds to NLRP3 in the cytoplasm and can trigger inflammasome activation. Xian et al. also discovered that different NLRP3 inflammasome activators can rapidly stimulate monocarboxylate transporter-mediated calcium uptake, thereby opening mPTP and triggering VDAC oligomerization. This process is independent of the mtDNA or ROS that induces the generation of Ox-mtDNA. Inside mitochondria, Ox-mtDNA is repaired by the DNA glycosylase OGG1 or cleaved by the endonuclease FEN1 into 500–650 bp fragments. These fragments leave the mitochondria through mPTP and VDAC-dependent channels to initiate cytoplasmic NLRP3 inflammasome activation. The above studies demonstrate that oxidized mtDNA activates the NLRP3 inflammasome. Additionally, in recent years, studies have indicated that mtDNA, as an activator of the NLRP3 inflammasome, may be implicated in several diseases, such as atherosclerosis, age-related macular degeneration, mevalonate kinase deficiency, and certain bacterial infections, signifying that mtDNA can serve as a disease-related inflammasome agonist [14, 60].

In recent years, mtDNA has become a research hotspot. Many studies have shown that mtDNA activates the NLRP3 inflammasome, but there are still many unresolved issues in the mechanism. First of all, up to now, no study has shown how mtDNA enters the cytosol, and the structural characteristics and sequences of immune-stimulating molecules are still unknown. Secondly, although some studies have shown that oxidized mtDNA can activate the NLRP3 inflammasome and mROS is necessary for the oxidation of mtDNA, the role of mROS in the activation process of the inflammasome is controversial, and ROS itself also has its specific signal transduction and even destructive effects [61]. Therefore, there are still many problems that need to be further overcome and improved in the process of mtDNA activating the inflammasome.

6. The NLRP3 inflammasome as drug potential for autoimmune diseases

The abnormal activation of NLRP3 inflammasome plays a key role in innate immunity. The abnormal activation of NLRP3 inflammasome is associated with various diseases such as diabetes, atherosclerosis, metabolic syndrome, cardiovascular diseases, and neurodegenerative diseases. Therefore, the study of potential inhibitors of NLRP3 inflammasome has important clinical significance. So far, studies have identified the direct inhibition of NLRP3, indirect inhibition of ASC, Caspase-1, IL-1 signaling pathways, and NLRP3 inflammasome-related signaling (**Figure 2**).

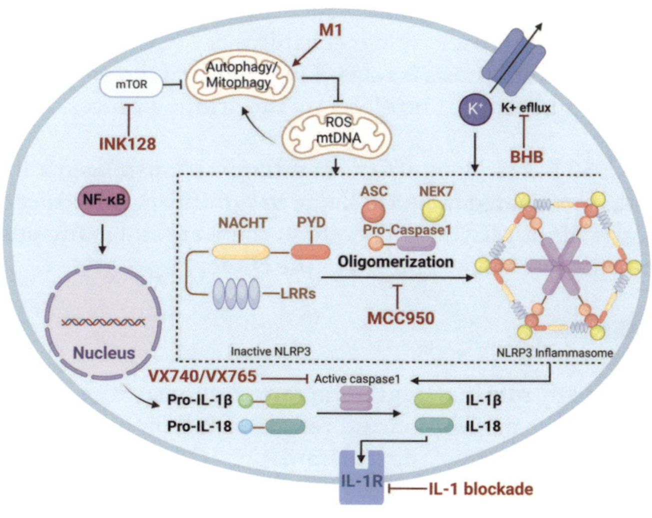

Figure 2.
Potential strategies for NLRP3 inflammasome inhibition. MCC950 inhibits the assembly of NLRP3 bodies by inhibiting NLRP3 oligomerization. VX740 and VX765 can inhibit activated Caspase 1. By blocking the downstream signaling pathway of IL-1, the release of IL-1 is inhibited. Inducing autophagy can remove inflammasome activators and degrade inflammasome components and damaged mitochondria to inhibit NLRP3 inflammasome activation. M1 inhibits NLRP3 inflammasome activation by inducing autophagy; mTOR is a negative regulator of autophagy, and INK128, as an inhibitor of mTOR, induces autophagy and inhibits NLRP3 inflammasome activation. BHB inhibits K+ efflux, indicating that regulating ion flow is also an effective strategy.

6.1 NLRP3 inhibitors

MCC950 is currently the most studied and most effective NLRP3 inflammasome inhibitor. It is a diaryl sulfonylurea compound [62]. It has high specificity and has no inhibitory effect on NLRP1, AIM2, and NLRC4. Its mode of action is to inhibit the activation of NLRP3 inflammasome and reduce the secretion of IL-1β by eliminating ASC oligomerization in human and mouse macrophages [62]. The mechanism of action of MCC950 includes directly interacting with the Walker B motif in the NACHT domain of the NLRP3 protein to block the hydrolysis of ATP, thereby inhibiting the activation of NLRP3 and the formation of inflammasomes [63]. MCC950 can inhibit the release of IL-1β induced by NLRP3 activators [64].

At present, many studies on MCC950 show that it has obvious effects in animal models of various inflammation-related diseases. For example, in a mouse model of spontaneous chronic colitis, by oral administration, it can significantly improve body weight, colon length, colon weight-to-body weight ratio, disease activity index, and histopathological score [65]. Moreover, it can significantly inhibit pro-inflammatory cytokines (such as IL-1β, IL-18, IL-1α, IFN-γ, TNF-α, IL-6, IL-17, chemokine MIP1a and NO) [66]. In addition, NLRP3 inflammasome is involved in the pyroptosis of macrophages. Pyroptosis is a pro-inflammatory cell death and is involved in the pathogenesis of atherosclerosis [67]. Zeng et al. [68] used $ApoE^{-/-}$ mice and ox-LDL-induced THP-1-derived macrophages MCC950 to treat the mechanism of atherosclerosis. MCC950 was intraperitoneally injected into 8-week-old $ApoE^{-/-}$ mice and fed with a high-fat diet for 12 weeks. THP-1-derived macrophages were treated with ox-LDL and MCC950 for 48 hours, respectively. The results showed that the plaque area and macrophage content in the MCC950 treatment group were reduced. However, in the in vivo study, the lipid profile of the aortic root of $ApoE^{-/-}$ mice was not improved. Zeng et al. [68] concluded through experiments that MCC950 can inhibit the activation of NLRP3 and GSDMD-N axis and reduce macrophage pyroptosis. And it was concluded that the anti-atherosclerotic mechanism of MCC950 inhibiting macrophage inflammation and apoptosis is related to inhibiting the assembly and activation of NLRP3 inflammasome and has no effect on the priming process of NLRP3 inflammasome activation.

Although MCC950 has obvious effects in inflammation-related animal models, its clinical trial was terminated in phase II due to significant off-target effects and toxicity in clinical trials of MCC950. Therefore, there are still many problems to be overcome before MCC950 can be applied in the clinic.

6.2 Caspase-1 inhibitors

Caspase-1 plays a key role in the inflammatory response. By activating inflammasomes, it can cause the maturation and release of inflammatory cytokines such as IL-1β and IL-18, thereby triggering inflammation. Currently, some common Caspase-1 inhibitors mainly include VX-740, VX-765 and oridonin. Among them, the widely studied ones are VX-740 and its analog VX-765, which are peptidomimetic inhibitors of Caspase-1 [69]. They can also block the cleavage of pro-IL-1β/18 by covalent modification of the catalytic cysteine residue in the catalytic active site of caspase-1 [69]. In addition, VX-740 has been proven to be able to reduce joint damage in rheumatoid arthritis (RA) and osteoarthritis (OA) in mouse models [70]. In phase I and II clinical trials for RA patients, it initially showed good therapeutic effects, but the research was forced to be suspended due to its hepatotoxicity [71]. VX-765 can also improve rheumatoid arthritis and psoriasis in mouse models by reducing the release of IL-1β and IL-18 [72]. However, Caspase-1 is still not applied in clinical applications.

6.3 IL-1 blockades

IL-1β and IL-18, as the main products of activated NLRP3 inflammasomes and potent pro-inflammatory cytokines, mediate the pathogenesis of many inflammatory or autoimmune diseases. Therefore, IL-1 blockade is also a feasible treatment approach for related inflammatory diseases. Currently, some common drugs used for IL-1 blockade include: anakinra and rilonacept. Anakinra is an IL-1 receptor antagonist that blocks the biological activity of IL-1 by binding to the receptor of IL-1. Anakinra has been approved worldwide for RA, SLE, adult-onset Still's disease (AOSD), and JIA [73–76]. However, anakinra has a short half-life and requires daily injection [77]. Rilonacept is a recombinant dimer fusion protein that blocks the signal transduction of IL-1α and IL-1β. It is used to treat cryopyrin-associated periodic syndromes, including familial cold autoinflammatory syndrome and Muckle-Wells syndrome. Several clinical trials have also shown that rilonocept is effective in treating gout [78–80]. In recent years, the IL-18 blocking antibody GSK 1070806 is in early development [81]. By blocking IL-1, these drugs can effectively improve the symptoms of inflammation-related diseases. At the same time, it may also cause some adverse reactions, such as an increased risk of infection. Therefore, the use of such drugs must be cautious.

6.4 Inhibition of NLRP3-related signaling pathways

The activation of the NLRP3 inflammasome can lead to the occurrence of inflammatory responses. Therefore, inhibiting the NLRP3-related signaling pathway has become a current research hotspot. Studies have shown that autophagy can induce NLRP3 phosphorylation and inhibit NLRP3 inflammasome activation by removing inflammasome activation stimuli and degrading inflammasome components [82]. The active metabolite M1 of ginsenoside becomes an inhibitor of the NLRP3 inflammasome by inducing autophagy [83]. In the mouse model of LN, the rapamycin target protein (mTOR) activates the inflammasome by inducing NLRP3 expression through ROS. At the same time, mTOR is also a negative regulator of autophagy. Inhibiting mTOR can induce autophagy, and autophagy can inhibit the activation of the NLRP3 inflammasome. Therefore, the mTOR inhibitor INK128 can be used as a treatment method for inhibiting NLRP3-related pathways [84]. In addition, the activation of the NLRP3 inflammasome can cause pyroptosis, which is involved in many pathological processes. Zhou et al. [85] conducted phenotypic screening of NLRP3-dependent pyroptosis and obtained a new compound N77. The biological target of N77 is glutathione-s-transferase Mu 1 (GSTM1). Its mechanism of action is that GSTM1 may regulate the glutathione modification of caspase-1 and may be a negative regulator in the activation of the NLRP3 inflammasome. And in the in vivo study by Zhou et al., N77 significantly improved the inflammatory response in the pyrothermal-related acute keratitis model, providing a new inhibitor of NLRP3 inflammasome-induced pyroptosis. Moreover, inhibiting the upstream signals of NLRP3 is also a feasible treatment method, for example, inhibiting K+ efflux, ROS production, and lysosome rupture to prevent the activation of the NLRP3 inflammasome. However, there is still a long way to go in clinical applications. In conclusion, there are sufficient research results indicating that NLRP3 is closely related to many autoimmune diseases. Therefore, it is imperative to develop more effective and less toxic inhibitors.

7. Conclusion

Mitochondria have long been regarded as the core hub of energy conversion within cells. However, its large and unique genome possesses the ability of immune activation apart from encoding essential proteins, enabling mitochondria to undertake multiple responsibilities in cells. Even though the endosymbiotic theory has not been fully confirmed, the phenomenon that mitochondrial genomes are detected by intracellular DNA sensors and trigger a series of inflammations inevitably leads to frequent doubts about its special identity. The large copy number of mtDNA and its vulnerable storage location also make one suspect that such an exquisite design must undertake responsibilities beyond encoding important mitochondrial proteins. In this article, we have reviewed that mtDNA, as an innate immune agonist, can trigger interferon responses and inflammatory responses by activating the cGAS-STING pathway and the NLRP3 inflammasome signaling pathway. MtDNA enters the cytosol due to mitochondrial homeostasis imbalance and mitochondrial DNA release caused by various intracellular and extracellular unstable factors, and there it comes into contact with the DNA sensor cGAS. The nucleotide transferase domain of cGAS forms a dimer after binding to the dsDNA backbone, thereby further catalyzing cGAMP and enabling it to perform the function of a second messenger, activating STING, and promoting its translocation to the Golgi apparatus to recruit TBK1 and IRF3. After further phosphorylating and activating IRF3, it enters the nucleus to exert its functions, triggering downstream ISGs and type I interferon responses, and inducing inflammatory effects. NLRP3 is similar. Mitochondrial dysfunction causes oxidized mtDNA to be released into the cytoplasm. Through the interaction of NLRP3, ASC, and pro-caspase-1, the formed inflammasome complex will cleave and generate active IL-1β and IL-18 and release them outside the cell, triggering inflammatory responses. After the signaling pathway mechanisms activated by mtDNA of cGAS-STING and NLRP3 are revealed, some possible new therapeutic targets for diseases involving innate immunity related to them have also been obtained. For cGAS-STING, the pathogenic mechanism of autoimmune diseases and the development of treatment regimens have new directions. The immunocheckpoint blockade therapy has new solutions in the predicament of its frustrated treatment efficiency. The development of targets related to the mtDNA release mechanism is also expected to play a greater role in fields such as tumor immunity. The development of NLRP3 inhibitors, Caspase-1 inhibitors, and IL-1 blockers, as well as drugs based on other targets of this pathway, has achieved significant results in the early theoretical studies. However, intracellular signal regulations often have non-single functions. For example, the cGAS-STING pathway can both promote the killing of T cells through interferon responses and upregulate the expression of PD-L1 to enhance the immune escape of cancer cells, making the drug development of this pathway unable to proceed with a single regulatory scheme. In studies of inhibitors targeting other targets of the NLRP3 signaling pathway, negative effects of varying degrees have also emerged, highlighting the complexity of the signaling pathway. However, scientists are also actively seeking solutions for example, under specific conditions, or combined with gene therapy to enhance the original therapeutic effect on tumors. Nevertheless, in general, the current mechanism of mitochondrial release is still unclear. If issues such as what determines its release mode and what its specific and effective contents are can be solved, perhaps starting from the upstream, the pathway of triggering the innate immune response through mtDNA can provide better treatment methods and therapeutic effects for related diseases.

Abbreviation

ACLY	Adenosine 50 -triphosphate citrate lyase
AGS	Aicardi-Goutières syndrome
AOSD	Adult-onset Still's disease
$ApoE^{-/-}$	Apolipoprotein E knockout
ASC	apoptosis-associated speck-like protein containing a CARD
ATP	adenosine triphosphate
CDNs	cyclic dinucleotides
CD-NTase	cyclic dinucleotide nucleotidyltransferase
cGAMP	cyclic GMP-AMP
cGAS	cyclic GMP-AMP synthase
Cxcl10	CXC chemokine ligand 10
DAMPs	damage-associated molecular patterns
DNA	deoxyribonucleic acid
dsDNA	double-stranded DNA
ETC	electron transport chain
FEN1	flap endonuclease 1
GSDMD	Gasdermin D
GSDMD-N	Gasdermin D N-terminal domain
GTP	guanosine triphosphate
HIF	hypoxia-inducible factor
HSV-1	herpes simplex virus-1
IFIT3	interferon-induced protein with tetratricopeptide repeats 3
IFN	type I interferon
IFN-γ	interferon-γ
IL-17	interleukin-17
IL-18	interleukin-18
IL-1α	interleukin-1α
IL-1β	interleukin-1β
IL-6	interleukin-6
IRF3	interferon regulatory factor 3
ISGs	interferon-stimulated genes
JIA	juvenile idiopathic arthritis
LN	lupus nephritis
LPS	lipopolysaccharide
MIP1a	macrophage inflammatory protein 1 alpha
mPTP	mitochondrial permeability transition pore
mtDNA	mitochondrial DNA
mTOR	mechanistic target of rapamycin
NACHT	NAIP (neuronal apoptosis inhibitory protein), CIITA (MHC class II transactivator), HET-E (incompatibility locus protein from Podospora anserina), and TP1 (telomerase-associated protein 1)
nDNA	nuclear genome

NF-κB	nuclear factor kappa B
NLRC4	nucleotide-binding oligomerization domain-like receptor family CARD domain-containing 4
NLRP1	nucleotide-binding oligomerization domain-like receptor family pyrin domain-containing 1
NLRP3	nucleotide-binding oligomerization domain-like receptor family pyrin domain-containing 3
NLRs	nucleotide-binding oligomerization domain (NOD)-like receptors
NO	nitric oxide
OGG1	8-oxoguanine DNA glycosylase 1
Ox-LDL	oxidized low-density lipoprotein
Ox-mtDNA	oxidized mitochondrial DNA
PAMPs	pathogen-associated molecular patterns
PD-L1	programmed death ligand 1
PRRs	pattern recognition receptors
RA	rheumatoid arthritis
RLR	RIG-I-like receptor
ROS	reactive oxygen species
SLE	systemic lupus erythematosus
STING	stimulator of interferon genes
STING CTD	STING C-terminal domain
TBK1	TANK-binding kinase 1
TFAM	transcription factor A, mitochondrial
TLR9	toll-like receptor 9
TLRs	toll-like Receptors
TNF-α	tumor necrosis factor-α
$Trex1^{-/-}$	three prime repair exonuclease 1 gene knockout
TRIM21	tripartite motif containing 21
VDAC	voltage-dependent anion channel
VSV	vesicular stomatitis virus

Author details

Yinghong He†, Boyuan Shen† and Xiang Zhou*
College of Life Sciences and Health, Wuhan University of Science and Technology, Wuhan, Hubei, China

*Address all correspondence to: zhouxiang@wust.edu.cn

† Yinghong He and Boyuan Shen contributed equally.

References

[1] Friedman JR, Nunnari J. Mitochondrial form and function. Nature. 2014;**505**(7483):335-343. DOI: 10.1038/nature12985

[2] Shadel GS, Clayton DA. Mitochondrial DNA maintenance in vertebrates. Annual Review of Biochemistry. 1997;**66**:409-435

[3] Shadel GS, Horvath TL. Mitochondrial ROS signaling in organismal homeostasis. Cell. 2015;**163**(3):560-569

[4] West AP, Shadel GS, Ghosh S. Mitochondria in innate immune responses. Nature Reviews. Immunology. 2011;**11**(6):389-402. DOI: 10.1038/nri2975. Epub 2011 May 20

[5] Weinberg SE, Sena LA, Chandel NS. Mitochondria in the regulation of innate and adaptive immunity. Immunity. 2015;**42**(3):406-417

[6] Ding C, Song Z, Shen A, Chen T, Zhang A. Small molecules targeting the innate immune cGAS-STING-TBK1 signaling pathway. Acta Pharmaceutica Sinica B. 2020;**10**:2272-2298

[7] Shimada K, Crother TR, Karlin J, Dagvadorj J, Chiba N, Chen S, et al. Oxidized mitochondrial DNA activates the NLRP3 inflammasome during apoptosis. Immunity. 2012;**36**(3):401-414

[8] Mishra P, Chan DC. Mitochondrial dynamics and inheritance during cell division, development and disease. Nature Reviews Molecular Cell Biology. 2014;**15**(10):634-646

[9] Supinski GS et al. Mitochondria and critical illness. Chest. 2020;**157**(2):310-322

[10] Collins LV et al. Endogenously oxidized mitochondrial DNA induces In vivo and In vitro inflammatory responses. Journal of Leukocyte Biology. 2004;**75**(6):995-1000

[11] Picca A et al. Cell death and inflammation: The role of mitochondria in health and disease. Cells. 2021;**10**(3):537

[12] Szczesny B et al. Mitochondrial DNA damage and subsequent activation of Z-DNA binding protein 1 links oxidative stress to inflammation in epithelial cells. Scientific Reports. 2018;**8**(1):914

[13] Lu P et al. Mitochondrial DNA induces nucleus pulposus cell pyroptosis via the TLR9-NF-κB-NLRP3 Axis. Journal of Translational Medicine. 2023;**21**(1):389

[14] Riley JS, Tait SW. Mitochondrial DNA in inflammation and immunity. EMBO Reports. 2020;**21**(4):e49799

[15] Zanini G et al. Mitochondrial DNA as inflammatory DAMP: A warning of an aging immune system? Biochemical Society Transactions. 2023;**51**(2):735-745

[16] Ning L et al. Cytosolic DNA-STING-NLRP3 Axis is involved in murine acute lung injury induced by lipopolysaccharide. Clinical and Translational Medicine. 2020;**10**(7):e228

[17] Pandey A et al. Cell biology of inflammasome activation. Trends in Cell Biology. 2021;**31**(11):924-939

[18] West AP, Shadel GS. Mitochondrial DNA in innate immune responses and inflammatory pathology. Nature Reviews Immunology. 2017;**17**(6):363-375

[19] Oduro PK et al. The cGAS-STING signaling in cardiovascular and metabolic diseases: Future novel target option for pharmacotherapy. Acta Pharmaceutica Sinica. B. 2022;**12**(1):50-75

[20] Riley JS et al. Mitochondrial inner membrane Permeabilisation enables mtDNA release during apoptosis. The EMBO Journal. 2018;**37**(17):e99238

[21] McArthur K et al. BAK/BAX macropores facilitate mitochondrial herniation and mtDNA efflux during apoptosis. Science. 2018;**359**(6378):eaao6047

[22] Cosentino K et al. The interplay between BAX and BAK tunes apoptotic pore growth to control mitochondrial-DNA-mediated inflammation. Molecular Cell. 2022;**82**(5):933-949.e9

[23] Newman LE, Shadel GS. Mitochondrial DNA release in innate immune signaling. Annual Review of Biochemistry. 2023;**92**:299-332

[24] Li J-Y et al. TRIM21 inhibits irradiation-induced mitochondrial DNA release and impairs antitumour immunity in nasopharyngeal carcinoma tumour models. Nature Communications. 2023;**14**(1):865

[25] Miao R et al. Gasdermin D permeabilization of mitochondrial inner and outer membranes accelerates and enhances pyroptosis. Immunity. 2023;**56**(11):2523-2541.e8

[26] Shokolenko I et al. Oxidative stress induces degradation of mitochondrial DNA. Nucleic Acids Research. 2009;**37**(8):2539-2548

[27] Ablasser A, Chen ZJ. cGAS in action: Expanding roles in immunity and inflammation. Science. 2019;**363**(6431):eaat8657

[28] Sun Z, Hornung V. cGAS-STING signaling. Current Biology: CB. 2022;**32**(13):R730-R734

[29] West AP et al. Mitochondrial DNA stress primes the antiviral innate immune response. Nature. 2015;**520**(7548):553-557

[30] Hu M et al. ATM inhibition enhances cancer immunotherapy by promoting mtDNA leakage and cGAS/STING activation. The Journal of Clinical Investigation. 2021;**131**(3):e139333

[31] Saffran HA et al. Herpes simplex virus eliminates host mitochondrial DNA. EMBO Reports. 2007;**8**(2):188-193. DOI: 10.1038/sj.embor.7400878

[32] Corcoran JA et al. Herpes simplex virus UL12.5 targets mitochondria through a mitochondrial localization sequence proximal to the N terminus. Journal of Virology. 2009;**83**(6):2601-2610

[33] Wassermann R et al. Mycobacterium tuberculosis differentially activates cGAS- and inflammasome-dependent intracellular immune responses through ESX-1. Cell Host & Microbe. 2015;**17**(6):799-810

[34] Wiens KE, Ernst JD. The mechanism for type I interferon induction by mycobacterium tuberculosis is bacterial strain-dependent. PLoS Pathogens. 2016;**12**(8):e1005809

[35] Watson RO et al. The cytosolic sensor cGAS detects mycobacterium tuberculosis DNA to induce type I interferons and activate autophagy. Cell Host & Microbe. 2015;**17**(6):811-819

[36] Collins AC et al. Cyclic GMP-AMP synthase is an innate immune DNA sensor for mycobacterium tuberculosis. Cell Host & Microbe. 2015;**17**(6):820-828

[37] Brokatzky D et al. A non-death function of the mitochondrial apoptosis apparatus in immunity. The EMBO Journal. 2019;**38**(11):e100907

[38] Aarreberg LD et al. Interleukin-1β induces mtDNA release to activate innate immune signaling via cGAS-STING. Molecular Cell. 2019;**74**(4):801-815.e6

[39] Wang C et al. Manganese increases the sensitivity of the cGAS-STING pathway for double-stranded DNA and is required for the host defense against DNA viruses. Immunity. 2018;**48**(4):675-687.e7

[40] Liu Z-S et al. G3BP1 promotes DNA binding and activation of cGAS. Nature Immunology. 2019;**20**(1):18-28. DOI: 10.1038/s41590-018-0262-4

[41] Dai J et al. Acetylation blocks cGAS activity and inhibits self-DNA-induced autoimmunity. Cell. 2019;**176**(6):1447-1460.e14

[42] Chu L et al. Perillaldehyde inhibition of cGAS reduces dsDNA-induced interferon response. Frontiers in Immunology. 2021;**12**:655637. DOI: 10.3389/fimmu.2021.655637

[43] Li S et al. The cyclopeptide Astin C specifically inhibits the innate immune CDN sensor STING. Cell Reports. 2018;**25**(12):3405-3421.e7

[44] Haag SM et al. Targeting STING with covalent small-molecule inhibitors. Nature. 2018;**559**(7713):269-273

[45] Thomsen MK et al. The cGAS-STING pathway is a therapeutic target in a preclinical model of hepatocellular carcinoma. Oncogene. 2020;**39**(8):1652-1664

[46] Lood C et al. Neutrophil extracellular traps enriched in oxidized mitochondrial DNA are interferogenic and contribute to lupus-like disease. Nature Medicine. 2016;**22**(2):146-153

[47] Giaglis S et al. Circulating mitochondrial DNA copy numbers represent a sensitive marker for diagnosis and monitoring of disease activity in systemic lupus erythematosus. RMD Open. 2021;**7**(3):e002010

[48] An J et al. Expression of cyclic GMP-AMP synthase in patients with systemic lupus erythematosus. Arthritis and Rheumatology. 2017;**69**(4):800-807

[49] Caielli S et al. Erythroid mitochondrial retention triggers myeloid-dependent type I interferon in human SLE. Cell. 2021;**184**(17):4464-4479.e19

[50] Quintero-González DC et al. Mitochondria as a key player in systemic lupus erythematosus. Autoimmunity. 2022;**55**(8):497-505

[51] Caielli S et al. Oxidized mitochondrial nucleoids released by neutrophils drive type I interferon production in human lupus. The Journal of Experimental Medicine. 2016;**213**(5):697-713

[52] Xiang W et al. Inhibition of ACLY overcomes cancer immunotherapy resistance via polyunsaturated fatty acids peroxidation and cGAS-STING activation. Science Advances. 2023;**9**(49):eadi2465

[53] Lang T, Lee JPW, Elgass K, Pinar AA, Tate MD, Aitken EH, et al. Macrophage migration inhibitory factor is required for NLRP3 inflammasome activation. Nature Communications. 2018;**9**(1):2223

[54] Kelley N, Jeltema D, Duan Y, He Y. The NLRP3 inflammasome: An overview of mechanisms of activation

and regulation. International Journal of Molecular Sciences. 2019;**20**(13):3328

[55] Kodi T, Sankhe R, Gopinathan A, Nandakumar K, Kishore A. New insights on NLRP3 inflammasome: Mechanisms of activation, inhibition, and epigenetic regulation. Journal of Neuroimmune Pharmacology. 2024;**19**(1):7

[56] Huang Y, Xu W, Zhou R. NLRP3 inflammasome activation and cell death. Cellular & Molecular Immunology. 2021;**18**(9):2114-2127. DOI: 10.1038/s41423-021-00740-6. Epub 2021 Jul 28

[57] Shi J, Zhao Y, Wang K, Shi X, Wang Y, Huang H, et al. Cleavage of GSDMD by inflammatory caspases determines pyroptotic cell death. Nature. 2015;**526**(7575):660-665

[58] Nakahira K, Haspel JA, Rathinam VA, Lee SJ, Dolinay T, Lam HC, et al. Autophagy proteins regulate innate immune responses by inhibiting the release of mitochondrial DNA mediated by the NALP3 inflammasome. Nature Immunology. 2011;**12**(3):222-230

[59] Xian H, Watari K, Sanchez-Lopez E, Offenberger J, Onyuru J, Sampath H, et al. Oxidized DNA fragments exit mitochondria via mPTP- and VDAC-dependent channels to activate NLRP3 inflammasome and interferon signaling. Immunity. 2022;**55**(8):1370-1385.e8

[60] Liu Q, Zhang D, Hu D, Zhou X, Zhou Y. The role of mitochondria in NLRP3 inflammasome activation. Molecular Immunology. 2018;**103**:115-124

[61] Xian H, Liu Y, Rundberg Nilsson A, Gatchalian R, Crother TR, Tourtellotte WG, et al. Metformin inhibition of mitochondrial ATP and DNA synthesis abrogates NLRP3 inflammasome activation and pulmonary inflammation. Immunity. 2021;**54**(7):1463-1477.e11

[62] Coll RC, Robertson AA, Chae JJ, Higgins SC, Muñoz-Planillo R, Inserra MC, et al. A small-molecule inhibitor of the NLRP3 inflammasome for the treatment of inflammatory diseases. Nature Medicine. 2015;**21**(3):248-255

[63] Coll RC, Hill JR, Day CJ, Zamoshnikova A, Boucher D, Massey NL, et al. MCC950 directly targets the NLRP3 ATP-hydrolysis motif for inflammasome inhibition. Nature Chemical Biology. 2019;**15**(6):556-559

[64] Vande Walle L, Stowe IB, Šácha P, Lee BL, Demon D, Fossoul A, et al. MCC950/CRID3 potently targets the NACHT domain of wild-type NLRP3 but not disease-associated mutants for inflammasome inhibition. PLoS Biology. 2019;**17**(9):e3000354. DOI: 10.1371/journal.pbio.3000354

[65] Perera AP, Fernando R, Shinde T, Gundamaraju R, Southam B, Sohal SS, et al. MCC950, a specific small molecule inhibitor of NLRP3 inflammasome attenuates colonic inflammation in spontaneous colitis mice. Scientific Reports. 2018;**8**(1):8618

[66] Bakhshi S, Shamsi S. MCC950 in the treatment of NLRP3-mediated inflammatory diseases: Latest evidence and therapeutic outcomes. International Immunopharmacology. 2022;**106**:108595

[67] Zhang L, Jiang YH, Fan C, Zhang Q, Jiang YH, Li Y, et al. MCC950 attenuates doxorubicin-induced myocardial injury in vivo and in vitro by inhibiting NLRP3-mediated pyroptosis. Biomedicine & Pharmacotherapy. 2021;**143**:112133

[68] Zeng W, Wu D, Sun Y, Suo Y, Yu Q, Zeng M, et al. The selective

NLRP3 inhibitor MCC950 hinders atherosclerosis development by attenuating inflammation and pyroptosis in macrophages. Scientific Reports. 2021;**11**(1):19305

[69] Cornelis S, Kersse K, Festjens N, Lamkanfi M, Vandenabeele P. Inflammatory caspases: Targets for novel therapies. Current Pharmaceutical Design. 2007;**13**(4):367-385

[70] Rudolphi K, Gerwin N, Verzijl N, van der Kraan P, van den Berg W. Pralnacasan, an inhibitor of interleukin-1beta converting enzyme, reduces joint damage in two murine models of osteoarthritis. Osteoarthritis and Cartilage. 2003;**11**(10):738-746

[71] Strand V, Sokolove J. Randomized controlled trial design in rheumatoid arthritis: The past decade. Arthritis Research & Therapy. 2009;**11**(1):205

[72] Wannamaker W, Davies R, Namchuk M, Pollard J, Ford P, Ku G, et al. (S)-1-((S)-2-{[1-(4amino-3-chloro-phenyl)-methanoyl]-amino}-3,3-dimethyl-butanoyl)-pyrrolidine2-carboxylic acid ((2R,3S)-2-ethoxy-5-oxo-tetrahydro-furan-3-yl)-amide (VX-765), an orally available selective interleukin (IL)-converting enzyme/caspase-1 inhibitor, exhibits potent anti-inflammatory activities by inhibiting the release of IL1beta and IL-18. The Journal of Pharmacology and Experimental Therapeutics. 2007;**321**(2):509-516

[73] Jesus AA, Goldbach-Mansky R. IL-1 blockade in autoinflammatory syndromes. Annual Review of Medicine. 2014;**65**:223-244

[74] Calabrese LH. Anakinra treatment of patients with rheumatoid arthritis. The Annals of Pharmacotherapy. 2002;**36**(7-8):1204-1209

[75] Kalliolias GD, Liossis SN. The future of the IL-1 receptor antagonist anakinra: From rheumatoid arthritis to adult-onset Still's disease and systemic-onset juvenile idiopathic arthritis. Expert Opinion on Investigational Drugs. 2008;**17**(3):349-359

[76] Dein E, Ingolia A, Connolly C, Manno R, Timlin H. Anakinra for recurrent fevers in systemic lupus erythematosus. Cureus. 2018;**10**(12):e3782

[77] Granowitz EV, Porat R, Mier JW, Pribble JP, Stiles DM, Bloedow DC, et al. Pharmacokinetics, safety and immunomodulatory effects of human recombinant interleukin-1 receptor antagonist in healthy humans. Cytokine. 1992;**4**(5):353-360

[78] Schumacher HR Jr, Sundy JS, Terkeltaub R, Knapp HR, Mellis SJ, Stahl N, et al. Rilonacept (interleukin-1 trap) in the prevention of acute gout flares during initiation of urate-lowering therapy: Results of a phase II randomized, double-blind, placebo-controlled trial. Arthritis and Rheumatism. 2012;**64**(3):876-884

[79] Mitha E, Schumacher HR, Fouche L, Luo SF, Weinstein SP, Yancopoulos GD, et al. Rilonacept for gout flare prevention during initiation of uric acid-lowering therapy: Results from the PRESURGE-2 international, phase 3, randomized, placebo-controlled trial. Rheumatology (Oxford, England). 2013;**52**(7):1285-1292

[80] Schumacher HR Jr, Evans RR, Saag KG, Clower J, Jennings W, Weinstein SP, et al. Rilonacept (interleukin-1 trap) for prevention of gout flares during initiation of uric acid-lowering therapy: Results from a phase III randomized, double-blind, placebo-controlled, confirmatory efficacy study.

Arthritis Care Research (Hoboken). 2012;**64**(10):1462-1470

[81] Ozaki E, Campbell M, Doyle SL. Targeting the NLRP3 inflammasome in chronic inflammatory diseases: Current perspectives. Journal of Inflammation Research. 2015;**8**:15-27

[82] Harris J, Lang T, Thomas JPW, Sukkar MB, Nabar NR, Kehrl JH. Autophagy and inflammasomes. Molecular Immunology. 2017;**86**:10-15

[83] Lin TJ, Wu CY, Tsai PY, Hsu WH, Hua KF, Chu CL, et al. Accelerated and severe lupus nephritis benefits from M1, an active metabolite of ginsenoside, by regulating NLRP3 inflammasome and T cell functions in mice. Frontiers in Immunology. 2019;**10**:1951. DOI: 10.3389/fimmu.2019.01951

[84] Li X, Zhang X, Pan Y, Shi G, Ren J, Fan H, et al. mTOR regulates NLRP3 inflammasome activation via reactive oxygen species in murine lupus. Acta Biochim Biophys Sin (Shanghai). 2018;**50**(9):888-896

[85] Zhou N, Zhang Y, Jiao Y, Nan J, Xia A, Mu B, et al. Discovery of a novel pyroptosis inhibitor acting though modulating glutathionylation to suppress NLRP3-related signal pathway. International Immunopharmacology. 2024;**127**:111314